This book was written thanks
to the unconditional support of my lover,
Marco B. I hope it will contribute
to creating a better world where my daughters,
Justine and Matilda, will be able to live
the life they choose to the full.

Stéphanie

Since I was a child, I have lived surrounded
by piles of books. I owe them my epiphanies,
and some have changed my life. I am very
grateful to have been able to create one of them
with care, love and patience. Thanks Eve,
Stéphanie and my mum.

Olympe

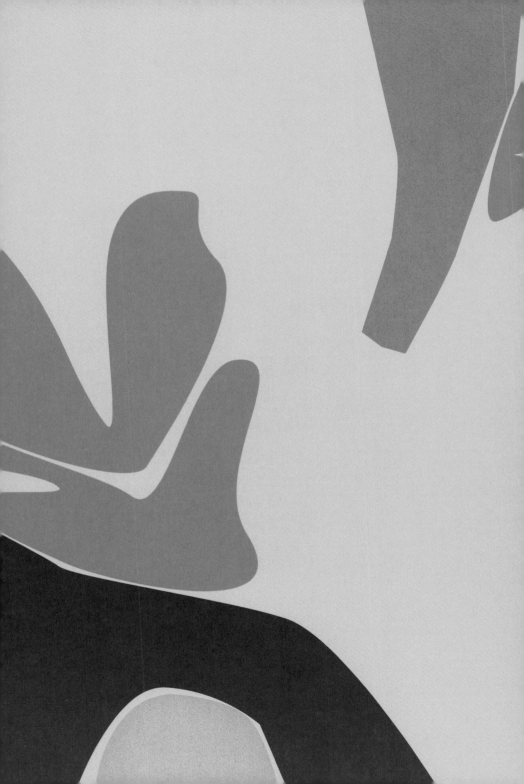

Sex Talk

A Feminist Discussion of Sexual Empowerment

Stéphanie Estournet
Olympe de Gê

Hardie Grant

BOOKS

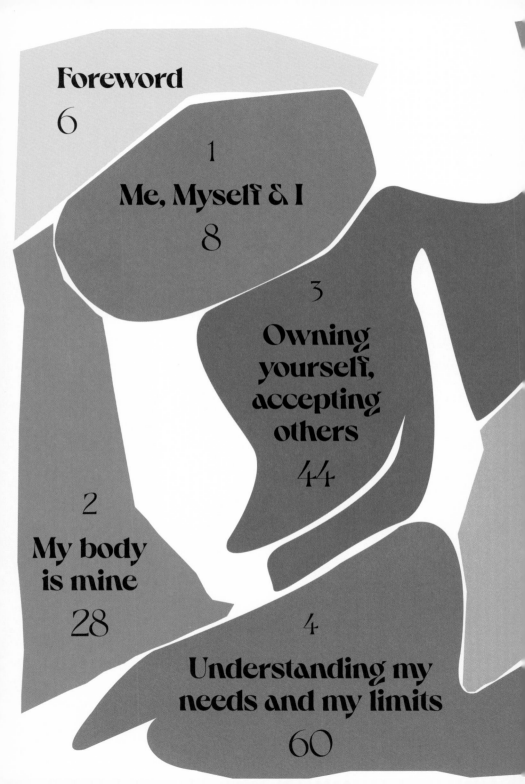

Foreword
6

1
Me, Myself & I
8

3
Owning yourself, accepting others
44

2
My body is mine
28

4
Understanding my needs and my limits
60

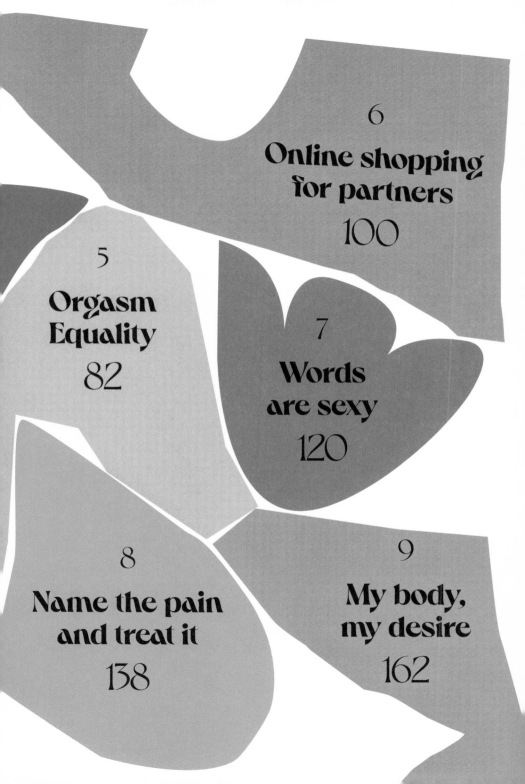

6

Online shopping for partners

100

5

Orgasm Equality

82

7

Words are sexy

120

8

Name the pain and treat it

138

9

My body, my desire

162

Foreword

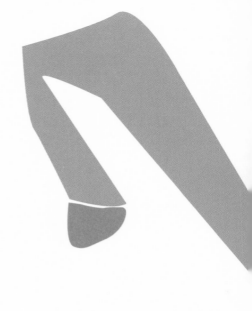

Olympe (O de G) Sex is political.

Stéphanie (SE) Do you really think so?

O de G During sexual intercourse, the man will probably orgasm; it's much less likely that the women will, however, don't you think? It's not an even playing field when it comes to pleasure. And that is political.

SE But in that case, wearing lingerie, shaving your body hair, going on a diet ... That's also political, right?

O de G Women have been brought up to give pleasure. Visual, sensual, sexual. We don't learn to take it freely. Neither do we learn to occupy space, our space. So yes, our bodies, what we do with them, are political.

SE We need to learn to know ourselves intimately.

O de G To live for ourselves first and foremost, beyond masculine validation.

SE To deconstruct the roles we've been assigned.

O de G To take hold of and develop what does us good.

This is how it all began. This is how Stéphanie Estournet and Olympe de Gê, two French women with very different viewpoints, began a series of discussions that went on to provide the substance of *Sex Talk*.

An author and journalist specialising in body representation and sexualities, Stéphanie Estournet is in a traditional heterosexual relationship with her lover, who is 'often more feminist than she is'. She has two daughters. She is convinced of the need to remain as closely attuned as possible to oneself, and to identify and deconstruct toxic models.

A militant feminist, Olympe de Gê set off down the road of pornography as a way of taking repossession of her body and her pleasure, and of demonstrating the beauty of bodies in their many guises. A performer in, and director of, several feminist pornographic films, she has since invested her skills in audio work, in particular by co-founding the inclusive audio-porn podcast *Voxxx*[1].

In order to write *Sex Talk*, Olympe and Stéphanie questioned experts, read dozens of fascinating books, and deconstructed (in part, at least!) their love lives. They engaged in multiple exchanges on social media, went to exhibitions, watched TV series and films, and discussed things over and over again, trying to work out concrete action plans to apply to our daily lives.

Sex Talk is aimed at all women, whatever their age and life journey, who wish to live outside the constraints placed upon them. Because before you share your pleasure and feelings, it helps to learn to know yourself and love yourself – in every sense of the word! *Sex Talk* offers a collection of thoughts on diverse subjects as well as recommending a wide variety of resources.

The aim is to enable each one of us to build a relationship with their body and their pleasure that, at long last, reflects their inner self.

| 1   voxxx.org

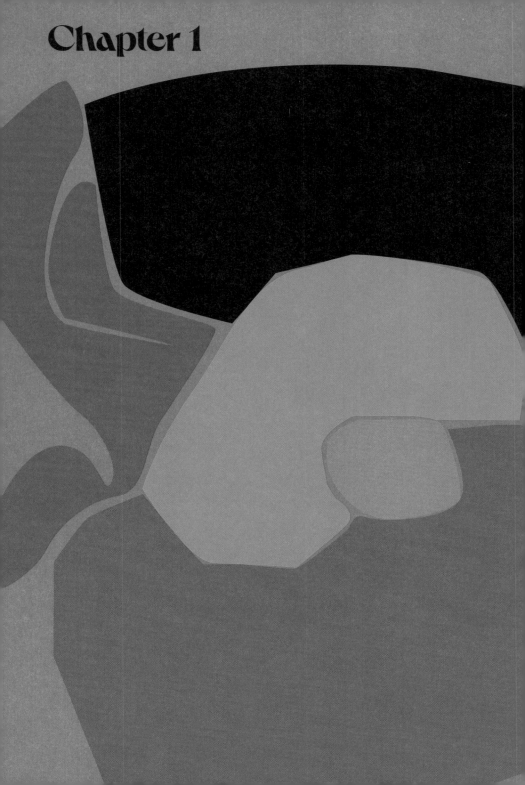

Chapter 1

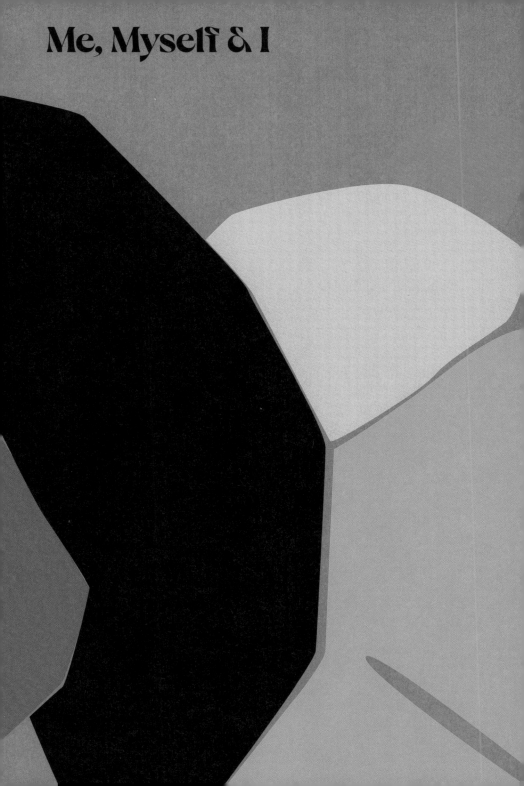

Me, Myself & I

The day we said to each other, 'OK, let's talk about sex – but let's really talk about it...'

'Is sexual pleasure really a political issue?' This question had been running through my mind since Olympe and I had left the flat in the Rue Louise Weiss, located in Paris's 13th arrondissement. There was a palpable sense of light-heartedness in the air that Saturday evening, in warm, post-lockdown June, as dusk languidly settled over the city. And the thought persistently looping through my brain was this: Are my orgasms and libido, my fantasies and pleasure, worthy of being pondered and publicly discussed, as is being advocated by post-#MeToo supporters? Those hands touching your buttocks on the underground or in the nightclub – something we've all experienced – do they reveal an ingrained sense of domination of one gender over the other? Is the push-up bra I'm wearing tonight proof that my body conforms to social control? And if I enjoy being spanked when playing erotic games, is this necessarily linked to how I relate to men?

There is, perhaps, something wildly indecent about discussing these topics publicly, but it's almost unavoidable in today's hypersexualised society. Given the constant exposure of eroticised women's bodies on screens, in public areas – indeed, everywhere I look – isn't it all too easy to be sucked into the performance and value-judgement aspects of matters that ought only to concern me and those close to me?

Are you alright? Olympe asks as we walk past the start-up campus, Station F.

It's been beautifully renovated, I reply, pointing to the glass-and-iron structure bathed in warm light.

Olympe smiles.

You're thinking about our earlier conversation? she asks.

Yes, I'm thinking about it. What's worse: I can't get it out of my head.

The evening began like so many other Parisian parties, as a low-key gathering in a friend of a friend's apartment: finding a kindred spirit, avoiding someone like the plague, standing there, holding an organic paper cup with your name on it, all to the soundtrack of a generic playlist.

When I go out to join her on the terrace, Olympe is surrounded by three women. Not girlfriends, as far as I know. I admire the spectacular view across to the François Mitterrand National Library and the Seine beyond it, and it takes me a moment to grasp that the tone of the conversation won't be to Olympe's liking.

I just don't understand why feminists feel the need to poke their noses into sexuality, intimacy. It's a couple's private life! says one thirty-something. I don't want to be lectured about what I get up to in bed.

I fake it; sometimes, I think I overdo it, jokes another. But seriously, if it makes him happy and I get to watch my series quicker, that suits me!

There are more important causes than sex if we want to fight for women's rights...

Like FGM, adds a third.

The women nod in agreement. The expression on Olympe's face is one of *Where is the nearest door to get the hell out of here?* There is always oppression that is more violent and worse than what we are experiencing, she begins. But isn't mentioning them a way of avoiding looking at what is happening in our own lives? So, for example, why do we force ourselves to make love? Why don't we feel able to simply say: 'No, I don't feel like it (any more)'? Marital duty is a thing of the past, isn't it?

Some people don't want to change; others are scared to do so...
We're now passing by a cinema, girls in crop tops and tracksuit bottoms are dancing to nineties hip hop. Guys sitting nearby look on and nod in time.

Don't be depressed, Olympe says. We both know there's still
a long, long way to go...

A tall blond guy throws an all-conquering look our way.

Hey girls, shall we go for a spin, me and your tight little butts? he calls.

Yes, there's still a lot of work to do, I tell Olympe. And I admit
that sometimes, I'm doubtful.

About what?

It's hard to explain. Olympe and I share the same values, more or less –
in short, anti-patriarchal, body positive and sex positive.

Women like those we met this evening, who give their guys
a blow job when asked. Who wear skirts because 'it makes
their man happy'. I sometimes ask myself if they aren't right.
Olympe laughs and looks at me. She thinks I'm joking. But I'm not.

That evening, one of the girls had told me about the lingerie she buys to look sexy when she makes her entrance – those were her words – into the bedroom. She likes to seduce her boyfriend, she likes the way he looks at her. She has a right to do so, doesn't she?

These questions on the basic tenets of the sex-positive positions adopted by me and Olympe often cross my mind. You only have to move away from feminist circles, and talk to women who haven't spent the past years discussing feminist issues in tight-knit groups, to be confronted by a completely different reality. And, more often than not, by a certain incomprehension of our outlook.

My work consists of observing and asking questions, and when something strikes me as dysfunctional or unfair, or where it seems possible to take such-and-such a step towards a happier life, I say so. As for questions about sexuality that liberate us, nothing is simple. And even if I am convinced of what I write – of the need to liberate our sexualities and our bodies – any counter-arguments make me stop and ask questions. They set alarm bells ringing. What if we're wrong – or, rather, what if we're not totally right? What if our truths only apply to a minority?

Caution and distance

Olympe and I met when, as a journalist, I got involved in her fundraising efforts to pay for the production of her first full-length film, *One last time*.[2] I'd been following her for a while; the first X-rated short film she'd directed, *The Bitchhiker*,[3] really fired me up, both physically and intellectually. It inverts the usual pornographic representations, and is anything but a textbook exercise: it's about a woman riding a powerful motorbike (played by Olympe herself), and the actors smile at and express their desire for each other. This left a lasting impression on me. Today, as I write these lines, I don't believe I'd ever seen a film before *The Bitchhiker* in which the actors expressed so much desire through their eyes. Over and above Olympe's militant approach as a director, her generous sincerity touched me to the core. Here was a woman with things to say, who had channelled to her advantage everything she had – from her artistic creativity (*The Bitchhiker* is, above all, a beautiful rather than an X-rated film) to her body – in order to be heard.

In 2021, we published our first joint work, *Jouir est un sport de combat*.[4] It comprised the diary of filming *Une dernière fois*, supplemented by Olympe's militant arguments. Working together allowed us to gauge the differences between our individual approaches. As an activist, and following a divorce, Olympe took control of her life as a woman – and of her sexuality – by performing in front of pornographer Lucie Blush's camera. She belonged to the Berlin queer scene, endured a barrage of online harassment and insults, and commenced a strike against heteronormativity.[5] When I think about it, I see a maelstrom of experiences, a series of shifting states – and also of pain. For my part, while sex has always played an essential role in my life, I have chosen to distance myself from it, to keep it inside my intimate sphere. At a very young age, I kept quiet on the subject. A girl who talked about sex in the 1990s was, for a heterosexual male, someone who could be cornered, who wouldn't say no. For other girls, she was a slut.

As a student, I worked as a freelancer on several pornographic magazines, inventing readers' letters; it was fun, a way of making a quick buck, and the workplace was respectful. I couldn't talk about my job to close friends and family, because I didn't want to make them feel uncomfortable. Later on, working for the daily newspaper, *Libération*, I wrote articles on sex. But there again, there was a degree of embarrassment at the heart of this 'progressive' publisher – not to mention my colleagues' lewd propositions.

Undeniably seventies...

I've often asked myself what it is that spurs someone to actively defend their ideas, or not to: *why* I didn't become an activist, despite some topics really getting under my skin. When discussing women's bodies and sexuality, there is a generational divide that needs to be considered. I was born in 1970. Just writing that down feels like a coming out, although it shouldn't be the case.

Today's thirty-somethings have taken up the torch of feminism and, as a corporatist reflex, they tend to stick with their own kind. A number of times over the last few years, I've felt out of place, different, even unwelcome. An older woman is supposed to make the most of herself in the eyes of her peers. She must be a model. After all, what's the point if all she provides is a reflection of what they don't want to see – an old woman?!

Believe me: it's hard to put up your hand in order to take the floor, and then tell a joke as an excuse for being so old. But I'm not trying to be like Calimero,[6] the odd one out (*such* a seventies reference), and it seems to me that if we want to understand our own motivations, we need to dig deep and analyse what we are today through what was handed down to us.

'President of the Republic'

Olympe grew up with her mother and sister; there were men around, too, but not on a day-to-day basis. In this world of women, she learned the need to be independent, especially from a financial perspective – a concept intrinsically linked to getting good grades at school and finding professional success. She likes to say, with a touch of humour, that when she became an adult, she was always the 'head of the family', taking the role of provider in the couples she formed. She paid the price for her spirit of independence. She's told me several stories about how much she suffered as an adolescent because she wasn't popular. She was two years younger, and head and shoulders taller, than the rest of her class, and, what's more, she didn't wear 'the right clothes'; she didn't have 'the right look'. And that's because her mother, who dressed her until she was in her teens, believed that her daughters shouldn't behave 'like sheep', whatever the personal cost.

In the same vein, her mother taught her that nail varnish, make-up and all these routines that women habitually follow, were a waste of time – time that could be utilised for more intelligent pursuits, such as 'becoming President of France'.

As for me, I was not brought up on the stereotypes for girls at the time. I didn't have any dolls (I didn't like them). I *was* taught how to do housework, but also, later on, how to do simple computer programming. I didn't wear a princess dress at Christmas, and found the witches in fairy tales much more appealing than the princes. A rounded education, you might think, except for the fact that I had a brother. And in the family hierarchy, he was everything. His father's son, the heir, hallelujah! If I had to stage this scene as a play, the girl would be somewhere in the shadows, barely distinguishable, while the boy would be busy getting up to 'boys' things; in the spotlight (he would gladly have given it a miss).

Perhaps things would have turned out differently if my mother, like Olympe's, had been affirmative, demanding and challenging. Instead, alongside her job as a teacher, she thrived in her roles as a 'good mother' and, as far as I know, a 'good wife' – the quotation marks here indicating the accepted norms of the 1950s and 1960s. I'm not bitter; I'm simply trying to understand.

Aged twenty-five, I had one regret: not having experienced flower power, a time of freshness, ripe with possibilities of change, new political standpoints and individual freedom. We had never been so free and equal. Images of Woodstock and the three Isle of Wight Festivals seemed like heaven: everyone was so peaceful, dancing semi-clad, kissing and sleeping on the ground in each other's arms.

It was as though this 'sexual revolution' could transform everything into a world of equality and love. Women challenged political and religious power. In the wake of major publications, such as *The Second Sex* by Simone de Beauvoir and Betty Friedan's *The Feminine Mystique*, women were uniting to demand their right to contraception and abortion – opening up the possibility of 'untrammelled' pleasure.[7] At last, they were taking ownership of their bodies! One thing I had missed, and only understood much later: history is written by those in charge. While women had more freedom, their relationship with men was still anything but equal. Men continued to take up all the available space, to occupy the highest platform on the podium, and to consider women as 'little helpers'. Don't they say that 'behind every successful man, there is a woman'?

What's more, while the times allowed women to more or less free themselves from religious and parental constraints regarding their sexuality, they also moved the goalposts: if you wanted to experiment and have sex experiences, you had to be a serial sexual adventurer, just like all-conquering men and their libidos. Being a 'liberated woman' became the new role to adopt in the company of men. But what about women for whom 'liberation' didn't involve their sexuality?

What about those women who were roused by this sudden moral freedom? Considering the patriarchy remained in charge, the urgency attached to sexual freedom often translated into making yourself available to a man and his pleasure, even at the risk of being considered a 'whore'.

Plenty of cultural objects from the 1970s evidence this mismatch, first up being Bernardo Bertolucci's film *Last Tango in Paris*, condemned at the time for its pornographic content but not at all for the violence perpetrated by the male character (Paul, played by Marlon Brando, forty-eight years old at the time) against the female character (Jeanne, Maria Schneider, nineteen years old). What shocked was the sex. The fact that a man violently subjugated a woman, in particular during the all-too-infamous scene of sodomisation, was not what was attracting any attention.

3am
Too fat, too thin, too hairy

What are you unsure about? Olympe continues, as we head towards the Seine. What makes you think it's sometimes better to force yourself to please others? I've done it; you've done it. Personally, I've even found myself pushing my own boundaries just to satisfy someone else's desires... And I got hurt! Don't you think it's healthier and safer simply to say: No, I don't want to?

I don't know. For me, when I have 'forced' myself, I didn't get hurt. And because I behaved like that for many years, I am convinced that being in a couple means compromise.

Olympe nods.

Compromises that we choose to make, you mean? she says. Or are the compromises imposed by men on us?

I'm not sure about that, I reply, somewhat dishonestly. But I guess it happens.

Olympe waits until we reach the middle of the walkway to pick up the conversation.

You can't live serenely if one person holds sway over the other, she says. If sex, which ought to be pleasurable, means that one person has rights and the other obligations. If you let yourself be drawn in when you're not in the mood, you can get hurt. And how does that make you look?

There's a lot of pressure...

Lots of different pressures, I'd say! Economic on all those women who are financially dependent on their partners; emotional because we can feel emotionally pressured and are prepared to do anything for the person we love – unfortunately, that's romantic love for you! But the main pressures come from the patriarchy. It's what we're taught: do things to please the man you love, invest in the relationship, in your couple; look inwards, even into your intimate sphere, while he invests in the public sphere, looking outwards.

After a pause, Olympe continues:

I've realised something: I can no longer tolerate placing demands on myself to please them. Too fat, too thin, too hairy, not enough sex appeal, not bold enough. Shit. All that's over. I want us to appreciate each other or else not at all. Do I tell a guy he's too hairy? That it would be nice if he made an effort to bulk up his shoulders, or that I don't like his style? I no longer want to ask myself, am I right for this role? And neither do I want any woman to ask herself that question. Imagine if that's how things stood, if we were equal.

But there is some pleasure involved in it all, isn't there? I play the role of a woman, I wear heels and lipstick. He protects me, opens the door for me and pays the restaurant bill. It's kind of cute if you think about it...

Olympe smiles.

I've never seen you dressed like a femme fatale, she says.

Come on, you know what I mean...

But do you really know what I mean?

Because I keep quiet, my mouth hovering between a grimace and a smile, Olympe carries on.

Do you know where we are right now?

Let me see. If I look around, we're between the François Mitterrand library, the Ministry of Finance, an enormous theatre named after a hotel chain, and the cinema complex in Parc de Bercy.

We are also on the Simone de Beauvoir footbridge. The author of *The Second Sex*.

But there is some pleasure involved in it all, isn't there? I play the role of a woman, I wear heels and lipstick

I love it when Olympe smiles with her eyes.

It's given me an idea, she continues. We could carry out a sort of survey. Try to bring some clarity to all these questions being asked about our sexuality and our relationship to the world.

About our bodies and our gender, too, I say, nodding. So many things have been spoken and written since #MeToo. Personally, it would help me make sense of it all. If I'm honest, all these words sometimes leave me feeling confused.

That would be the objective. Let's make some decisions. Let's talk to some experts. To people who don't look like us, individuals who have taken other routes through life. We're white, you're in your fifties, I'm in my thirties; let's meet up with women of colour, trans women, sex workers. Young women, older women. And get together with some male allies, too. Let's start reading, look around us and compare the fruits of our research.

The Paris lights were twinkling along the banks of the Seine, and there were hardly any passers-by. In the distance, even the hum of traffic seemed to have quietened. For me, as for so many Parisians, each area of the city has its own character, its own beauty, sometimes bound up with my own narrative.

We could arrange to meet up, I say. We could go for walks.
And share our findings and our thoughts.

I was seduced by the idea. Olympe is someone I know to be both very curious and very demanding when choosing which cultural products to be involved with. And we would be meeting women who would open our eyes to many issues.

As we walked the rest of the way across the bridge, our ideas snowballed: we could meet sex workers to gain insight into their thoughts and experiences; we could invite women and experts to join us on our walks; we could bring together artists' visions on these issues, the ones we're facing today and those from the pre-#MeToo era; we could explore comic books, TV series, art in the broadest sense of the term...

I smile, thinking of this project opening up before us: like two Penelopes riding out on their Odyssey.

Shall we start the ball rolling straight away?
Let's.

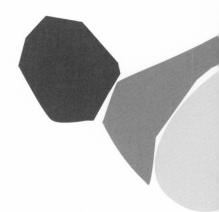

2   Gê (de), O. 2020, *One Last Time* – Olympe's first full-length film.
3   Gê (de), O. 2016, *The Bitchhiker*, Erika Lust Films.
4   Estournet, S. & Gê (de), O. 2021, *Jouir est un sport de combat*, Larousse, Paris.
5   *Olympe de Gê*, https://olympedege.com/blog/ – Olympe's blog (in English and French).
6   *Calimero*: a French cartoon character, is an unlucky little duck.
7   We are appropriating one of the most well-known slogans from May 1968: '*Vivre sans temps mort, jouir sans entraves*': 'To live instead of devising a lingering death, and to indulge untrammelled desire.' It is the last sentence of a situationist pamphlet, written by the Tunisian activist Mustapha Khavati in 1966.

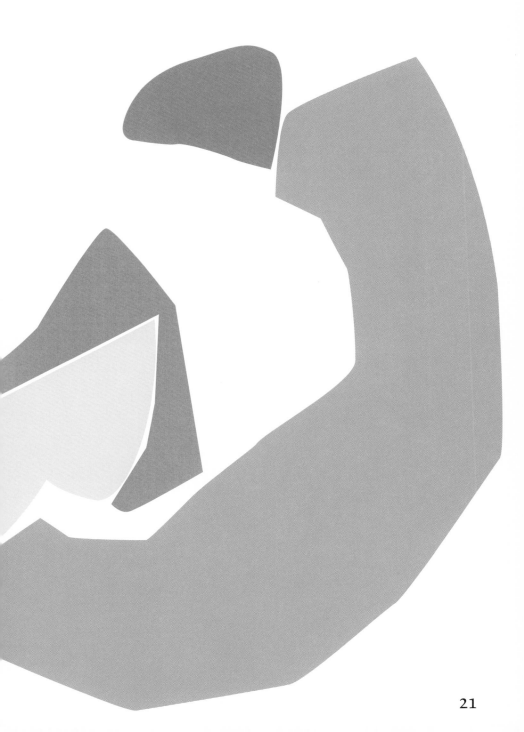

Marie Kirschen

'Herstory: looking at history from the female perspective for a change'

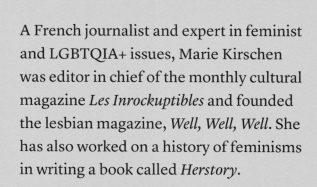

A French journalist and expert in feminist and LGBTQIA+ issues, Marie Kirschen was editor in chief of the monthly cultural magazine *Les Inrockuptibles* and founded the lesbian magazine, *Well, Well, Well*. She has also worked on a history of feminisms in writing a book called *Herstory*.

Olympe de Gê (O de G)   Your book, *Herstory*,[8] offers a social, political and popular ABC guide to different types of feminism. Even the title is a play on words, calling out how women have been overlooked in the way history has been written.

Marie Kirschen (MK)   Since time immemorial, history has been written by men. I don't know how things were for you at school; for me, the only women I heard about in my history lessons were queens and regents. The men were experts, artists, scientists, philosophers – they were *everything*.

O de G   An androcentric bias that erased women.

MK   There's one anecdote that I find especially revealing on this topic. It concerns the well-known anthropologist Claude Lévi-Strauss, when he was carrying out ethnographic observation of the Bororo, an indigenous people of Brazil. Back in 1936, Lévi-Strauss tells the following story: 'The whole village left the next day in around thirty canoes, leaving us alone with the women and children in the abandoned houses.'

SE   'Leaving us alone with the houseplants and the goldfish.'

MK   Spot on. What Lévi-Strauss is saying is that on the one hand, there are those who count – the men – and on the other, everyone else! It took until the 1970s before activists called out this androcentric approach, and gradually a space worthy of the name was given to women.

O de G   That was also when the militant writer Robin Morgan used the term 'herstory' to talk, at last, about history from women's point of view.

MK   Robin Morgan highjacked the word 'history' or, rather 'his story' to create the term 'herstory'. We tend to say that feminists don't have a sense of humour. Clearly that's not totally fair!

SE   Up to the present day – according to female observers – there have been three or four waves of feminism...

MK   Some male and female observers even go so far as to talk about *five* waves, adding a new wave for each generation. This representation has been criticised because it gives the impression that nothing happened during the first wave (1850–1945). And that nothing happens between each of them, which of course is false. It also fails by focusing only on what is happening in the West.

O de G   Each of these feminist waves has a distinct leitmotiv...

MK   The first wave took off in the mid-nineteenth century in Europe and the United States. Women were fighting to obtain civil and political rights. In 1893, New Zealand organised the first election in the world in which women participated. German and British women went to the polls from 1918 onwards; American women from 1920. In France, we had to wait until 1944 before French women were able to express their opinions through the ballot box.

O de G   Once they had gained their civic rights, women could finally embark on the question of the freedom of their bodies and their sexuality...

MK   Yes, and question the patriarchy and the traditional social model that, until that moment in time, had been imposed as the only acceptable norm: life as a housewife bearing children. The second wave mushroomed from the 1960s onwards in the United States, and in Europe from the 1970s. In France, women activists were demanding the right to do whatever they wanted with their bodies, in particular in matters of sexuality and terminations of pregnancy. The right to an abortion came into force in 1975. Other demands centred on housework being properly recognised.

SE   When we think that fifty years ago, women choosing to have an abortion were risking their own lives *and* criminal proceedings![9]

O de G   And then came the third wave...

MK   In 1992, the American activist Rebecca Walker – daughter of the writer Alice Walker, best known for her book *The Color Purple* – laid out her demands in an article in *Ms.* magazine: 'Becoming the Third Wave.' After civic rights and the right to do as one wishes with one's own body, it was time for feminist movements to really grapple with the specifics of racialised, transgender, lesbian women...

O de G   And that's when we start talking about intersectionality...

MK   Precisely. But we need to explain how this word originated on the militant scene.

SE   I've got a vague memory of a young Black lawyer talking about intersectionality for the first time when discussing discrimination suffered by Black women. It was in the 1980s, wasn't it?

MK   Yes; the lawyer you're referring to, Kimberlé Crenshaw, got involved in a case dating back to 1976 brought by American women against their employer, General Motors, on the grounds of unfair dismissal because they were *both* women *and* Black. In a substantial article (fifty or so pages long),[10] Crenshaw proved that American legislation presented a legal void, in that the victims suffered from several discriminations. With regards to the Black employees v General Motors case, discrimination as a woman was admissible, and so, too, was discrimination as a Black person, but not both. And yet a Black woman didn't have access to jobs for Black people, which were reserved for men, nor to jobs for women, which were reserved for white women.

O de G   It's a terrible story.

MK   As we're talking about discrimination, we could mention the discrimination affecting lesbian women, including within feminist movements. In France, for example, the Mouvement de Libération de la Femme, or MLF [Women's Liberation Movement], founded in 1970, tended to airbrush out lesbians, ordering them to stay in the closet. It even appeared at times to be homophobic or biphobic.

SE   I sometimes get the impression I don't understand anything about the history of feminism. Why can't women support each other? Does it depend on having a common form of teaching? Or sharing a culture – historical texts, for example? Even though I write *on* and *for* women, I confess I've never read *The Second Sex* by Simone de Beauvoir.

MK   Well, one to add to your reading list! [*laughter*] At the time, *The Second Sex* was extremely poorly received. It was 1949, and 'all the fuss and bother kicked up by females' was apparently over. After all, they'd got the vote – what else could they possibly want? Beauvoir called into question the notion of the very essence of a woman. In doing so, she anticipated gender studies. She asserted the right to abortion, and spoke out against the obligation of childbearing. She spoke about the body, the clitoris, the vagina, which caused an almighty scandal. Attacked on the right, and by some on the left who deemed her 'vulgar', her modern and foundation-laying words would be fundamental for many women from the MLF. With Simone de Beauvoir, everything changed!

O de G   What would you recommend we read?

MK   There are dozens of titles... The first that springs to mind – you'll certainly know it by heart – is *King Kong Theory* by Virginie Despentes. Published in 2006, this short book has cult status and is unusually powerful! Starting with experiences from her own life – including her rape, aged nineteen, and also her career as a sex worker – Despentes exposes the mechanisms adopted by the patriarchy. Her punchy writing turns it into a contemporary feminist manifesto. It's the sort of book you read and read again...

And I have a certain fondness for *Fun Home: a Family Tragicomic*, the graphic novel by Alison Bechdel. The author depicts her childhood, discovering herself, a growing awareness of her homosexuality, and her relationship with her parents, especially her father (who himself had homosexual relationships), weaving together a family mythology punctuated by numerous references to pop culture, Greek mythology and literature.

Lastly – but it's only what comes into my head, as there are so many works that deserve a mention – *Bad Feminist*, by Roxane Gay. This is an unashamed reflection on what it means to be a feminist. Yes, we are all riddled through with contradictions. And yes, you can shave, paint your nails, love pink and still condemn discriminations against women. As a bonus, it's beautiful writing, which never goes amiss!

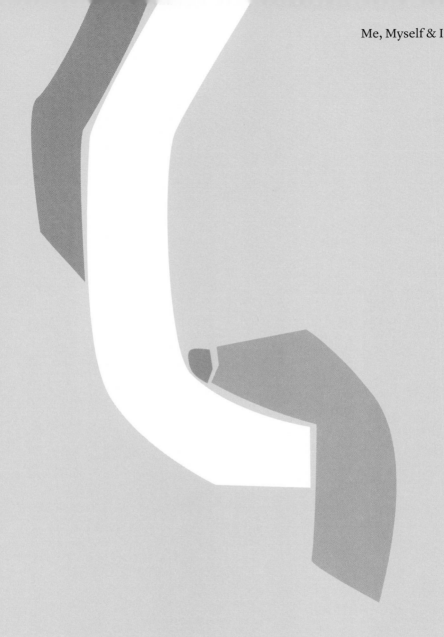

8   Kirschen, M. 2021, *Herstory, Histoire(s) des féminismes,* Edition la Ville Brûle, Paris.

9   At the time of writing, more than twenty American states have planned to ban abortion, some of which also plan to penalize it heavily. With the repeal of Roe v. Wade in 2022, the USA has gone back fifty years.

10 Crenshaw, K. 1991, 'Mapping the Margins: Intersectionality, Identity Politics and Violence against Women of Color,' *Stanford Law Review*, vol. 43, no. 6.

Chapter 2

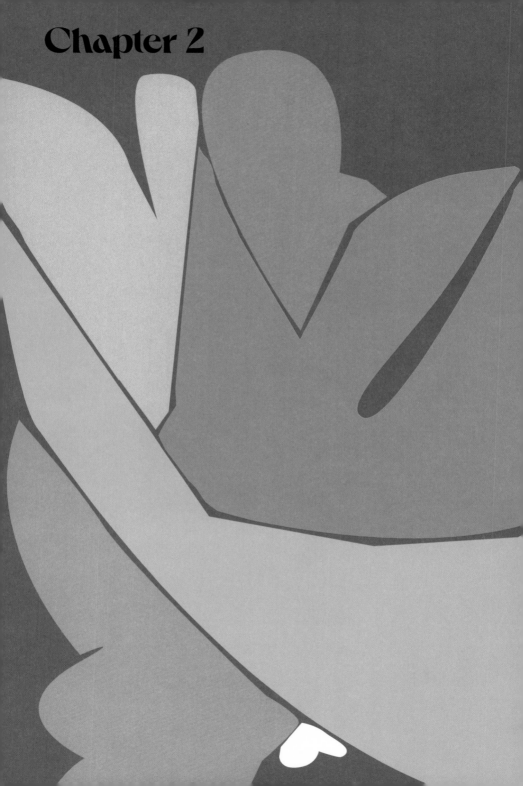

My body is mine

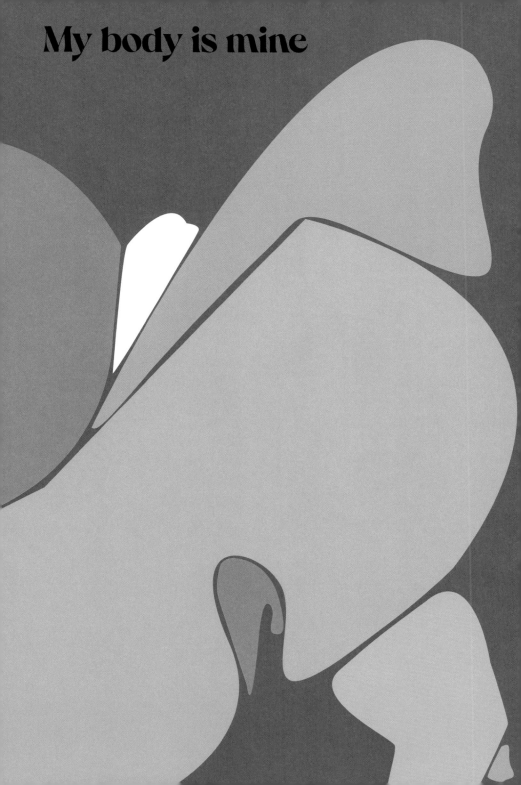

Sunday 18 July 2021

11am

Let's start with one of my favourite things in life: immersing myself in my books – those that, potentially, touch on the issue we're considering today with Stéphanie. I spread them around me in my bed – friends with whom to have a heart-to-heart. As mistress of ceremonies, I hand the floor to each of the authors. You first, Camille: remind me of how your relationship with your body has evolved since adolescence. And you, Gabrielle: tell me once again how difficult it is for you to go out and about in the world, to become a 'target', because your body is large. Éloïse, can you recall how you ended up appearing topless and why? And Virginie, how you reclaimed your body following a rape?

The patriarchy is a machine of rules and regulations dictating what we should do with every centimetre of our women's bodies. From our figures, the colour or texture of our hair, our skin, through to the shape of our breasts, the labia of our vulvas. A hierarchy is at play; it determines the best of the best, the most desirable and acceptable, then the 'bare minimum', and continues right through to the unacceptable. Where do these diktats lead us? Which medal are we supposed to win at the end? And most of all, what happens to us if we don't want to play along, or if we find ourselves at the bottom of the hierarchy?

Tuesday 20 July 2021

9.30pm

Today, Stéphanie and I had our first walk to discuss the topic of female empowerment. And we took the opportunity to go back to one of Paris's temples of the female body: the hammam at the Grand Mosque. I hadn't been there for absolutely ages, and yet, like in Paul Verlaine's poem, 'After Three Years': 'Nothing is changed, I see it all once more.' It is just as enchanting as I remember it, with its tall, tiled rooms and peaceful tempo, a place where everyone can enjoy a moment of tranquillity. 'Girl time, with no inhibitions,' enthuses a young woman, clearly there with her mother.

After the hammam, Stéphanie and I were quietly lying down in the vast relaxation room when a group of girls we'd noticed earlier – in their twenties and rather boisterous – sat behind us. After a few minutes, we started hearing them giggling... One whispered a little louder than the others, and I heard distinctly: 'She's King Kong's wife!' The others burst out laughing. Other women in the hammam frowned at them reproachfully, but I couldn't help turn red. I knew from their first sniggers that it was my – unshaved – legs and armpits that the girls were making fun of. We ignored them, but as soon as we arrived in the changing room, Stéphanie exploded:

What a violent comment! was her outraged reaction.
They can't just stick to things that concern them; they have
to judge and censure what other people choose to do.

I shrugged my shoulders.

It's a great opener for a discussion of the issues at hand, I said.
I don't think there is anything more divisive than body hair.

Even after lockdown, do you think? I've had the opportunity
to check a study on epilation in France. Since COVID, women
have adopted new habits: they are shaving less often.

I stroke my calves with the tips of my fingers.

Yet body hair remains unacceptable on a woman, I answer
fatalistically. Especially if said woman wants to be desirable. But
to be honest, I'm fed up to the back teeth of having to run through
this endless list of what I should be doing in the bathroom in order
to be desirable as a woman. Eyebrows, hair, body hair, nails, make-up.
Not to mention the cost of seeing a beautician and all the products
you have to buy to fix yourself up and fit in. Because that's what
it's all about, isn't it? Physically conforming to what is expected of us.

Stéphanie pouts:

Do you really believe that our obsession with eradicating body
hair is a marker of the patriarchy? That each and every chick
has assimilated some sort of standard, setting out that in order
to be desirable, you have to be hairless apart from on your head –
well, except for you?

Notes on various readings: why is body hair an object of such hatred?

I gently stroke my legs with a smile on my face. Body hair is one of those
issues that is obvious, because it affects all of us, regardless of gender,
and yet one we find hard to decode. While studying history of art, I was
confronted by representations of women in Western art who were readily
portrayed in all their voluptuousness, yet without body hair – zero, not
even a suggestive shadow. And what's more, I don't recall any teacher
ever daring to allude to this issue! Right back as far as ancient art, through
to Raphael's *The Three Graces* (1504–1505) and Giorgione and Titian's
Venuses (1510 and 1538), art has *only* depicted hairless women. We had
to wait until the nineteenth century for things to shift. The heroine
of Delacroix's painting *Liberty Leading the People* (1830) shows little more
than a suggestive hint of body hair under her armpits – yet she is evidently
a woman of the people, judging by her muscular build. In his 1866 painting
L'Origine du monde Gustave Courbet chose to portray a woman's genitals
with pubic hair – because he wanted to 'blow the lid off academic art',
explains Thierry Savatier,[11] a nineteenth-century art historian. In the
twentieth century, it was a combination of marketing and fashion that drew
attention to body hair. Gillette brought out its first women's razor in 1915
('The underarm must be as smooth as the face.'). Skirt lengths rose from
the 1920s onwards. Many widows were forced to go to work in the aftermath
of the first world war and enjoyed greater freedom. Fashion reflected this.
Skirts and dresses of the time revealed women's calves and even knees.

Razor manufacturers and producers of other shaving 'powder' products rubbed their hands with glee. Their recipe for success was simple: women have a problem (body hair); they have the solution.

With the arrival of pin-up girls, in particular the actress and singer Betty Grable – whose legs were insured for a million dollars – and the proliferation of fashion shoots, the result was a foregone conclusion: a 'real' woman doesn't have armpit or leg hair. From the 1970s onwards, when mini-skirts and bikinis became the norm, body hair was removed from every nook and cranny. Creams, wax, sugar, tweezers, thread... Just thinking about the fact that we're sold on the idea that hair removal is 'me time' makes *my* hair stand on end...

I'm not alone in not removing my body hair (which is a great comfort), if I can believe the initiatives launched by artists and models. In 2014, the photographer Ben Hopper caused a stir around the world with his 'Natural Beauty' project, depicting young women (performers, students, artists) with full armpit hair. Many women today choose to let their body hair be. And some celebrities show themselves in public, fuzz and all. Such a display is still *highly risky*. Take, for example, the model Arvida Byström, who, after posing for Adidas sporting hairy legs, wrote on Instagram on 25 September 2017: 'Me being such an abled, white, cis body with its only nonconforming feature being a lil leg hair. Literally I've been getting rape threats in my DM box. I can't even begin to imagine what it's like to not possess all these privileges and try to exist in the world.'

Thursday 22 July 2021

8pm

Having a drink with Marie,[12] in a sun dress, sublime in her new body.

2.45am

This sentence about Marie...

I was intending to write about our moment together – nothing special, in truth. And then I suddenly found myself judging my friend as being 'gorgeous' because she'd shed twelve kilograms. I couldn't stop thinking about it all evening. And now, it's almost 3am. I have to get up in the morning and I can't rid myself of the nagging in my head from my monkey mind.[13] My monkey mind accuses me of hierarchising beauty according to weight. Of not deconstructing the patriarchal conditioning I'm calling out – the fact, for example, that a beautiful woman should be slim and young.

My monkey mind tells me I am a usurper – just like the others, in fact – and that my feminist posturing doesn't stand up to scrutiny.

Why was I so pleased for Marie? Is it because she'd lost weight, because she had a body that 'conforms'? Fat phobia is extraordinarily widespread. It can be detected from a very young age: almost 50% of girls aged 3 to 6 are afraid of being fat! As a lot of people, I have had a fat phobic bias. I remember wishing I wasn't sitting next to that fat person on the plane. I remember making fun of my very chubby neighbour who lived in a 10m^2 studio. I remember loving Wall-E. I remember adding 'fat' before 'dumb', as if that were worse. And then I also had fat phobia towards myself. While my body is within the norm, I blamed myself a lot when I gained 5, 10 kilos, I did drastic diets, I hated myself.

But I have become aware that losing weight is not necessarily good news, far from it. It can reveal a deteriorating physical health, or mental health. Being slim doesn't mean being in good health. For women, a sudden weight change may be a sign that she is experiencing domestic violence. In Marie's case, she broke up with Mehdi. A few weeks later, she said she wanted to get back her life, and 'spring-clean from ceiling to floor'. During what she envisaged as a thorough spring-clean, she went to see a dietician regularly and started a diet. We didn't see each other for a while due to work. And now here she is, radiant, comfortable in her own skin.

I'd never seen Marie happy in her own skin (or not to this extent). I think that's where the issue lies. I'm happy for my friend. Not because she'll be able to fit into a size-ten bikini this summer, but rather because she set herself a challenge and is delighted to have achieved it. Had she lost two kilos, or none at all, or gained twenty more, it would have been the same for me, providing she was happy in herself.

Another friend, Soline, gained confidence by practising body building at a high level. Her muscular V-shaped back amazed me. As for Ursula, a friend from high school, blonde and thin, very tortured ... I saw her again 10 years later. She had gained 50 kilos. And she was glowing! She had opened an Instagram account on which she posted pictures of her naked body. She had many fans. She had never been so fulfilled, for the simple reason that she had finally succeeded, through a long therapy, to tame her anorexia. She had gained weight, and was alive, fat, amazing! And, fun fact ... Ursula also posted on her Instagram account close-ups of her boob hair ... and her mustache!

Friday 23 July 2021

11.35am

Stéphanie is epilating. She says she finds it more attractive, that she feels great when she leaves the beauty salon. In contrast to the girls she mentioned the other day, at the Grand Mosque, for whom hair removal is linked to being eligible in a man's eyes (a 'Prince Charming' – Walt Disney, get the hell out of our lives!), Stéphanie talks about her relationship with her body. Does this mean that she is ready to conform with what she thinks she needs to do with her body hair as a woman? Or should we conclude she has gone beyond this point and untangled all the exhortations, and today simply does whatever she wants?

In 2021 in France, 56 per cent of women aged under twenty-five stated they removed all their pubic hair. A significant trend when you realise that this figure rose by 11 per cent between 2013 and 2021. The same study[14] confirmed that 57 per cent of male and female respondents were bothered by hairy women's legs.

Have I ever felt 'bothered' by another person's body hair? Or by any other traditional marker of masculinity and femininity that goes against the grain? A couple of years ago, I was bowled over by the story of Harnaam Kaur, a young British girl who has polycystic ovary syndrome that manifests itself, amont other signs, in excessive hairiness. In every sense a 'girl', with her well-defined eyeliner, ornate piercings and scarlet lipstick, Harnaam Kaur also sports a thick, full black beard – not peach fuzz.

My adolescence was synonymous with experiencing great difficulty fitting in. I didn't understand the codes. I had always been the 'beanpole', the girl who sat at the back of the class to keep out of the way. Skeletor, daddy-long-legs, flat as a pancake... I heard it all. On reading about Harnaam Kaur, I couldn't begin to imagine her distress, aged eleven, at having to wax her body two or three times a week. The teasing, the insults. Can you imagine trying to be cool when you are the girl with the beard at a time when conventions tell us you have to epilate right down to those three hairs on each toe?

I looked at Harnaam Kaur's photographs on her Instagram account.[15] In her shoes, would I have had the courage to choose to present myself as she has done? To call on us to celebrate 'our individualities' and those things about ourselves that we criticise as 'flaws'? To encourage each and every one of us to be 'ourselves'?Things change – get better. I showed some photos of Harnaam Kaur to a friend's sixteen-year-old daughter. 'Oh, she's wearing a lot of make-up,' was her first reaction. Followed by: 'What a beautiful piercing.' And lastly: 'Her beard looks so soft.'

7pm

Cancelled this evening's date. I've got my period. Don't feel like it.

Sonia, whom I met in Berlin, and who is now working for a classified ads website, told me the other day that her firm provides sanitary products free of charge in its lavatories. 'They think of them on a par with loo paper, and you don't bring that to work with you, so why should it be any different for sanitary stuff?'

I was blown away.

'Red alert', 'the curse', 'the time of the month'... Periods remain a sort of punishment mixed with shame. We are in pain and worried about leaks. And even about being seen as a girl on her period, as though it is some kind of disability. Perhaps one day, through encouraging people to talk about it, by playing down the whole issue, we will stop being scared of leaks and stains (a fear we experience, on average, five days per cycle, which means sixty-five days a year!); we will no longer feel dirty on the grounds that our body odour changes; no longer worry about the reaction of guys if we're out on a date – precisely – or if we soil the sheets. Perhaps, lastly, as for Sonia and her company, sanitary products will be paid for by society as a whole, and we can put an end to menstrual insecurity.

'On average, having periods costs over €5,000 over the course of a lifetime. [...] This is about basic products that should be free or reimbursable.'[16] While I'm talking statistics, around 500 million people with vulvas suffer each year from menstrual insecurity, while 100 million youngsters miss up to one week of school each month because they have no access to sanitary protection.[17] If municipal, regional and local authorities, or the Ministry for Education, could earmark a tiny fraction of their budgets to address this problem, it would be a step towards equality.

Sunday 25 July 2021

5pm

Sipping an iced tea in the shade of my sweetgum tree, with my dog Mov at my feet and a number of books to hand in preparation for the next guest meeting Stéphanie and I have organised. Back to Paris this week. I'm not exactly looking forward to it.

I realise the extent to which I hide myself when I'm on my period. Not only because I feel ill. No, there's something more overarching. An unspoken pressure whispering in my ear: 'Deal with it! Your stomach hurts, you're feeling depressed: are these reasons to behave like a wimp? Be proud! Be strong!'

But... *why*, at the end of the day? Why do we feel the need to lick our wounds in secret each time we get our period? Why aren't we able to say to our bosses: 'Listen, you know what, I've got my period today and I just can't do it'? There's also pressure that we bring to bear on ourselves. That, along with our upbringing, and reinforced by society on a daily basis, amounts to a woman needing always to be at the top of her game.

I've been trying to rid myself of this pressure for a while now.

I've been trying to listen to myself first and foremost.

My body hair, my periods, my wrinkles, my weight... They are mine. Up to me to choose, according to my own feelings, how I want to navigate them. My choice as to what does and doesn't suit me. Not that it implies having to go on the offensive and shoot down in flames all those women and men who don't go along with it. I will just say very little: 'No, I'm not going to epilate. It's my body and I get to choose.' Or else, 'I've got my period, I don't feel great, I'd prefer to be on my own. I hope you understand.' If those at the other end don't understand, I'll make an effort – I promise! – to explain it again. But at the end of the day, as regards my body, the decisions are mine.

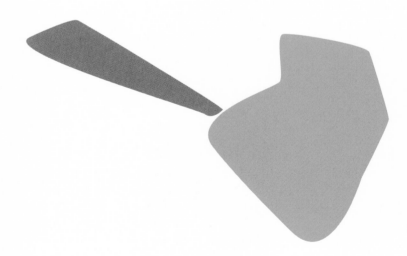

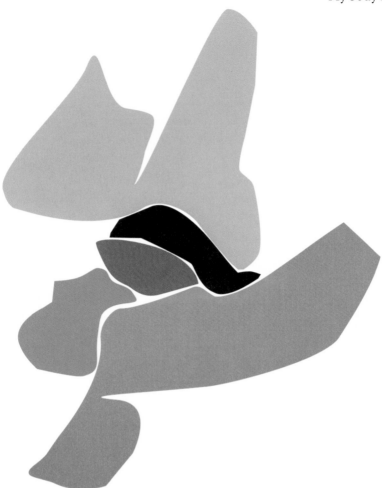

11 More can be found in: Savatier, T. 2009, *L'Origine du monde', histoire d'un tableau de Gustave Courbet*, Bartillat, Paris.

12 First and family names of individuals have been changed.

13 My monkey mind is an expression that encompasses all the confused states in which I find myself when everything gets muddled and I feel guilty, incapable, unstable and the victim of an injustice. And also unable to reflect clearly on things or let them go. I've borrowed this psychological metaphor from Chinese philosophy. It seems particularly fitting when I'm lying in bed in the middle of the night, chewing over a sentence I wrote the previous day!

14 2021, 'Le retour du poil, vers le fin de diktats?' *Ifop* (https://www.ifop.com/publication/le-retour-du-poil-vers-la-fin-des-diktats/).

15 @harnaamkaur, Instagram (https://www.instagram.com/harnaamkaur/).

16 Boston Women's Health Book Collective, The. 2011, *Our Bodies, Ourselves,* ninth edition, Simon & Schuster, New York.

17 According to the main French association that fights against period insecurity, Règles Élémentaires.

Going further

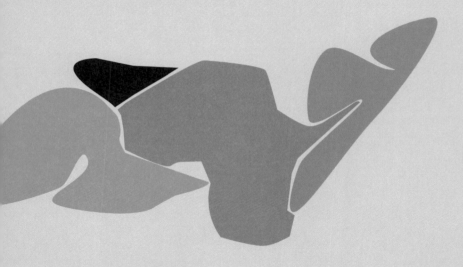

Discussions between friends, reactions on social media... Sexuality and our relationships with our bodies are finally coming into the open. Yet institutions still struggle to play their part in terms of information and education, and a taboo still hangs over the ways we talk about it. Until such time as sexuality and our relationships with our bodies really become topics like any others, here is an initial selection of resources to help put an end to conditioning and hidebound ideas about our bodies.

Megan Jayne Crabbe, *Body Positive Power*

Also known as Bodyposipanda, Megan Jayne Crabbe is a radiant representative of the body-positivity movement. Brainwashed from a very early age by the prevalent cult of thinness, she spent her entire adolescence wanting to be slimmer, slimmer and SLIMMER! Her body was the main stumbling block to her happiness: she would only be happy if she achieved the 'ideal weight'. This ultimately led her to a period of anorexia, bulimia and other eating disorders (EDs). One day, she asked herself: What if our bodies aren't the problem, but rather the way we are taught to perceive them? This provided her with a route to recovery – and to fat-positive activism! Megan Jayne Crabbe lives in the UK, from where she shares her feminist vision on a daily basis on Instagram, in a way that is inclusive and motivating. Her book, *Body Positive Power: How to Stop Dieting, Make Peace with your Body and Live*, is full of tips to help us love ourselves each day and deconstruct the norms. She dreams of a world in which all bodies are represented and celebrated, where the 'bikini body' diktat hasn't been invented, and where 97 per cent of women do not hate their body shape.

Essie Dennis, *Queer Body Power*

To what extent do the norms of beauty become overwhelming when one is not only fat but also queer? Does the body-positivity movement also represent people who can't be categorised using conventional gender expression? In *Queer Body Power*, Essie Dennis takes a radically deconstructivist approach to the idea of the 'perfect body', and wages war against the feeling of always being too *this* (too heavy, too masculine to be non-binary) or too *that* (too feminine to be lesbian, too fat to do drag). This book, with its powerful testimony and honest advice, opens up a fundamental conversation on body image and mental health from which LGBTQIA+ people are too often excluded.

Sonya Renee Taylor, *Your Body is Not an Apology Workbook*

What would our lives look like if we were free from the shame and fear of our own bodies? If we reached a state of radical love for ourselves? The author, poet and Black activist Sonya Renee Taylor likes to say that 'radical self-love is contagious [...]. You can totally catch it like a cold, but so is body shame, you know, and the truth of the matter is, we live in a world where we're constantly passing on body shame, all the time. And so if we're going to be contagious either way, I figure I might as well be spreading some radical self-love.'

This workbook, written in the wake of her bestselling book *The Body is Not an Apology*, asks you to 'draw, colour, doodle, talk to friends, take risks and perhaps step outside of what feels like your natural gifts and talents.'

Lena Dunham, *Girls*

Girls was a sensational series. In it, Lena Dunham displays her curvy body, without any retouching, including in sex scenes. When the series began, it was 2012 and curvy girls were still being asked to stay out of sight. Through scathing humour and realistic intimate scenes, we get to know Lena, a young woman who is not in touch with her own body, and finds it difficult to find her pleasure and express consent.

Since 2012, Lena Dunham has continued to write and regularly takes to Instagram. She has put on weight and her appearance has, of course, been commented on, and even vilified. Here is her public response:

When will we learn to stop equating thinness with health/
happiness? Of course weight loss can be the result of positive
change in habits, but guess what? So can weight gain.

Pussy Riots, 'Straight Outta Vagina'

We needed a period hymn. Since its inception in 2011, the Russian punk activist group Pussy Riot is famous for its feminist political outbursts and actions. 'Straight Outta Vagina' should be played at maximum volume!

Rupi Kaur, *Period*

Photographer, poet, producer, dancer – Rupi Kaur is a feminist artist of multiple talents. In 2015, she celebrated the beauty of periods in a series of photographs depicting bloodstained sheets in a washing machine, blood in a toilet bowl and a sanitary towel in a bin. The most famous of these images is of Rupi stretched out on her bed. Her sweatpants are bloodstained around the buttocks, and her bedsheet is, too. Instagram banned this photo twice... That sent it viral. Rupi Kaur castigated misogyny and the taboo surrounding periods. 'I bleed every month to help make humankind a possibility [...]. But a majority of people, societies and communities shun this natural process.'

Esther Calixte-Béa, @queen_esie

A committed activist from Montreal, Esther Calixte-Béa wants to normalise female body hair. Armpit hair, leg hair, chest hair, belly hair... She flaunts her hairiness with panache, extolling its beauty with a fashionable twist. Fed up with hating her body, she realised her complexes were damaging her mental health, and recognised the importance of working on the way we see our bodies. In 2021, the UK edition of *Glamour* dedicated its front page to her. She said: 'When I was a kid, I would have loved to see women like me, who showed off their hair [...]. I'd never seen a woman with chest hair on the cover of a magazine before. And it's me! I never thought I could make a difference and help change people's mentality!'

Chapter 3

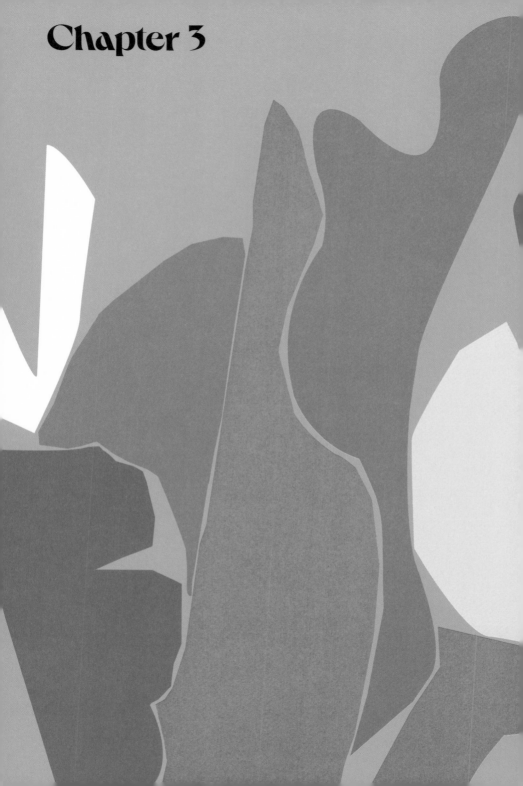

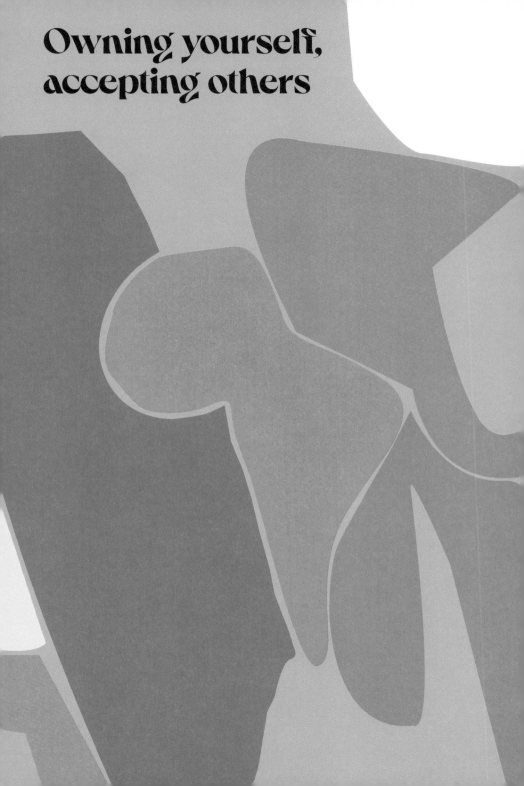

Owning yourself, accepting others

'A sex shop run by women.'

That's the goal of today's walk, suggested by Olympe. I didn't look the place up on Google; I prefer to find out about it in situ.

It's my old-school side: when someone mentions 'sex shop', my head fills with images of shelves of DVDs with hardcore sleeves, rows of flesh-coloured dildos, a range of crotchless French maids' outfits, all displayed under a harsh white light. When I was a student, I lived in Pigalle, at the time a diverse district where veteran Parisians would chat with prostitutes showing off their wrinkled cleavages while huge coaches disgorged their cargoes of tourists in search of 'seedy Paris' – with its golden-age cabarets, the prospect of fixed-price sex and, lurking behind heavy red curtains across doorways, its sex shops, where everything seemed to be allowed.

I found it absurd to be living in Pigalle without knowing what the place was all about. I couldn't afford to see a show at the Moulin Rouge or any of the cabarets in the area; I wasn't especially attracted to prostitutes; so all that remained were the sex shops. Even they were not something I was particularly inclined towards, but I thought I would try something new.

One afternoon, I decided I would push aside one of the red curtains and enter. I was alone – whether through being judgemental or indifferent, none of my friends would have come along. Sex shops at the time were the haunt of lonely perverts, men out on the town or depraved couples – 'normal' people were urged to find sexual satisfaction in the privacy of their own homes.

I'm not sure what I was expecting – at least something unusual, an amusing diversion. Music was blaring out of a radio; there was a smell of detergent; customers glanced around furtively; the guy working at the till was absorbed in reading his thriller. Nothing conjured up any hint of excitement or even disgust. There were, indeed, flesh-coloured dildos that brought a smile to my lips, arranged by size on a shelf a bit like a shooting range (and I had no idea they could be so *big*). Otherwise, there was nothing exciting about the place. I was disappointed.

Beautiful lighting and hipster assistants

I walk at Olympe's side along the narrow pavements in central Paris, and enjoy watching the motley crowd around us: families of tourists licking ice creams, gangs of teenagers with multicoloured hair, couples walking hand in hand...

Have you ever gone into one of those love shops? Olympe asks me, pointing at the midnight-blue façade of a boutique.

I went out of curiosity once or twice. People had harped on so much about them, and I wanted to understand how pre-millennium sex shops that were frequented by pariahs had transformed themselves into places to be, artfully nestling between a clothes shop and beauty products store.

The commercial side of things is savvy and the marketing slick. You can buy all sorts of sex toys, geisha balls, lingerie, as well as board games, and lubricants. These are all arranged in enticing stores that are properly illuminated and staffed by hipster assistants. The decor is designer, with no images of the naked body to be seen at all.

Isn't it a bit odd to hide the naked body when you're selling products linked to sexual pleasure? I muse.

Olympe smiles.

If it helps some people take their first step to discovering what they like, then why not? she says. Personally, I'm in favour of anything that gives people the key to pleasure!

Masturbation: to build yourself and find your pleasure

Further down the street, now that the traffic has died down, we spontaneously lower our voices; we definitely don't want our conversation to make anyone feel uneasy.

I don't recall exactly when I first started exploring my body, but I was young, continues Olympe. I had a sexuality of my own for years before I started experimenting with a partner. Today, I look back at that time as one of the most important stages in my sexual development. I know better what I do and what I don't like.

I was lucky enough to have had a very similar experience, I say. However, many girls remember being convinced as teenagers that masturbation was shameful. Some of them came from families who harped on at them that the Lord would punish them. Others were rapped over the knuckles if they so much as mentioned their vulvas, and so learned that the topic was dirty. They believed that the whole world would discover their 'guilty pleasure'.

Olympe nods her head in frustration.

Shame, the best way to straight-jacket us... she says.

Do you think you can learn about your own pleasure as an adult?

Better still, I believe you can learn it at any age.

I think that it also comes down to context, I say. Say, for example, that you split up from a toxic individual, you move to live somewhere that suits you better, you finally go on holiday; that means you'll be sleeping better, digesting better, and holistically be more in touch with yourself. If you're not having to put up defences in a hostile environment and can set aside time for yourself, the whole picture changes. You can be more in tune with your body.

And with what turns you on.

Olympe abruptly stops. Look, there it is, she says.

Across the road, we see a shop with a stylish wooden façade. In the window, subtly lit, are mannequins wearing sexy, 1920s-style clothing: short dresses with plunging necklines, long gloves that come up over the elbow, fringed baby-dolls in see-through lace...

How magnificent, I whisper.

The first part of the shop is spacious and inviting to wander around, reminiscent of the stores of luxury fashion designers. You move from a rail of sexy clothing to an arrangement of jewellery, including sensual items, all tastefully laid out to display the finest articles, using velvet cloth, marble plinths and tall, luxurious bamboo plants in large stone pots. The ambiance is plush without being remotely stilted. Behind the till are two women, one dressed in a dark suit and white trainers, the other wearing large-framed, pink-lensed glasses. They turn to greet us.

When I lived in Berlin, says Olympe, while eyeing up the leather harnesses, one of my friends suggested I wear one of these to meet my lover. She had a whole collection of them: for the waist, torso, breasts. I kind of wanted to but I didn't dare. She insisted that I would look amazing; it made me even more shy. But the idea made its way in my head. So one day, while she was cooking us lunch, I stuffed one into my bag. Not to steal it from her, but to try it out alone, without her trying to convince me. To make my own opinion.

You mean alone? Back at yours?

Yes. I waited until I was on my own and tried it on. I looked at myself wearing it for long minutes. I thought I didn't look bad. I looked great. Looking at myself in the mirror put me in the mood. A while later, I surprised my lover with it. He went crazy and I, too, felt amazing and in tune with myself. I also felt a sense of pride, as though I'd done something I didn't believe I was capable of doing.

I get it. Now that we're discussing it, I think that if someone suggested I wear a sexy outfit I'm not used to, or put on some jewellery, like those BDSM collars or maybe some nipple covers (look, there are several designs there made of black velvet shaped into hearts, thunderbolts and crosses), I would first want to get the hang of it *on my own*. To see whether I could play that role and feel at ease.

Learning to know yourself: self-pleasure and protection

When I was living in Pigalle, I wore red lingerie at the request of a boyfriend. For this guy – and for the times – it was somewhat transgressive: only pros wore that sort of underwear. I'd put the items on before going to meet him. I'd felt in disguise, older, out of place: this red lace simply wasn't me. I'd played along, before shoving the whole collection to the back of my wardrobe as the trappings of 'a bad girl'.

That can't have been very pleasant, sympathises Olympe, when I tell her the story.

That episode turned out alright. However, as for most of us, there were times of loneliness, when I would be crying my eyes out on my bed, disgusted with myself because I felt like I'd made a wrong choice. That I'd let myself be dragged into doing things to please a guy, unable to just say no, or explain that I didn't feel like it. Olympe nods.

These sorts of experiences can be really traumatising, she says. And there's no one-size-fits-all solution that you can systematically apply to avoid it happening... But let's go back to what we were saying just now about learning to know yourself, to understand what turns you on when you're alone. Not that it provides the key to unlock every situation, but it does allow you to listen more carefully to yourself when it comes to deciding whether to give some new experience a go. Don't you think?

We've moved through into the second room, which has grey glittery walls. The young woman in pink glasses is arranging a bamboo plant to the sound of catchy techno.

Please ask if you need any advice or information, she says.

There are sex toys for every shape and size, strap-ons, nipple-stimulators, straps, rigid ball gags... The space is entirely given over to them, arranged like works of art. Olympe is really taken by some fetish ballet shoes that keep your feet on tiptoes, thanks to 18-centimetre stiletto heels.

You have to learn to know yourself... she says. But also to accept yourself. I have always been very tall, and had a huge complex about my height. I was systematically put in the back row of any class photo. I was taller than the boys, while the norm is that a heterosexual girl must be shorter than her partner.

And even sufficiently short that she can wear heels and still not be taller than her beloved.

Behave like a girl, leaving him to play the 'heavyweight' – that's just it. I've lost count of the number of men around whom I've ended up concertinaing my hips, stooping to offset the couple of centimetres I've 'taken' from him... And then, gradually, I learned to accept my height. Taking pictures of myself and having friends photographing me certainly allowed me to be proud of it.

And that's exactly what countless people whose bodies do not conform to the norm do on social media: by taking photos of themselves and being complimented by well-meaning people, they learn to live not by dreaming of another body but by re-appropriating their own body. Happy in my skin, I can then turn my attention to the question of pleasure – no longer in connection with the other person and the pleasure I should be giving them, but pleasure for myself. The sort of enjoyment *I* want to feel. And that's essential.

Alone but well-equipped

A hand-embroidered leather strap-on hanging on the wall attracts my attention. I ask if I can take it down: it's a very beautiful piece, handmade by a Parisian craftswoman. The assistant explains how each of her pieces is individually designed – 'They can even be personalised.' We are a world away from the sex shops concealed behind red curtains and their rows of graduated flesh-coloured dildos! I wait until the assistant has moved away before returning to our conversation:

So, to recap, the first step, in your opinion, is to stop feeling sorry for not having a 'bombshell' body, and instead to learn to find yourself beautiful, sensual and desirable.

Exactly.

Step two: discover what you enjoy sexually outside time spent with a partner.

Olympe grins and gestures towards 'the most powerful vibrator in the world'.

Alone but well-equipped!

Is there a third step? I ask.

Of course, but we can start by concentrating on these two – by fantasising about... these two!

Olympe points to a gorgeous book displayed on a shelf. Two men are posing on the cover. They are joint winners of the first 'bombshell' body prize, but, more importantly, they are both wearing lingerie.

Not traditional boxers or leopard-print briefs. No. These guys are flaunting themselves in all seriousness and with flair, dressed in lace, their suspenders hanging down from their shirt tails, bound up in corsets and sporting black stockings.

I love it, exclaims Olympe. Don't you?

I don't know. I find it disorientating. These men are clearly very good-looking, but I can't help wondering how I would react if my partner showed up in suspenders . To be honest, I think I'd find it really difficult to deal with. I purposely avoid Olympe's question, asking one of my own:

What's left for us women if guys start wearing lace?

Olympe tries on a *Peaky Blinders*-style leather cap.

They're not stealing anything from us! Skirts, lingerie, trousers, make-up... Today, everyone should feel able to look however they want, adopt what suits them in their everyday lives – and in their intimate lives, too. We're heading in that direction, I think. And probably, in a few years' time, we'll be hanging out with blokes who dig out their best suspender belt to go on a date.

She's moved on from the cap, and is playing with a pair of fringed chaps. I know she's right. However, the idea continues to unnerve me.

Do you think masculine and feminine will disappear? I ask.

I think our masculine and feminine sides will be able to be expressed more and more freely, she says. In our private lives, as well. I hope so, in any case!

Be confident...

Of my height, my big nose, my flat chest ... of my masculine side, of what makes me feel good, beautiful.

Nail varnish: who is it for?

One day, my friend Max, a straight Italian with an ultra-masculine look and style, asked me for nail-varnishing tips. He seemed perfectly at ease with this idea, and once I'd got over my surprise, I showed him my nail varnish collection and offered to give him a manicure. At the end of the day, there was nothing odd about this lovely guy painting his nails. It was his body and he could do what he wanted with it. And what's more, the results were very rock 'n' roll and sexy.

An enormous plus for me, I think, is never having read women's magazines. It left me floundering, of course, because I didn't understand the references made by the girls around me. Besides, I didn't have many girlfriends. Boys, on the other hand, were cool with me once I'd got things straight with them: no, I'm not going to bed with you; treat me like an equal and don't play the super-hero – I can manage perfectly well on my own, thank you very much.

Today, I still find 'girlie things' difficult. I don't wear those pretty little bits of jewellery that come in gift boxes, and I know nothing about 'anti-ageing skin products' or what 'this season's fashion trends' are. Following in the footsteps of my grandmother, who did her nails while watching opera on VHS cassettes, my nails are always varnished. I like my hands to look well cared for. I often hear that a true feminist shouldn't be bothered about such things – putting on make-up, looking after her hands. But I think it comes down to what *I* like, and my ideas about my person generally suit me better than other peoples' ideas. So why is it so hard for me to accept that a man can be sexy dressed in lace?

Eventually we leave the shop, empty-handed. There's a storm in the air: it's humid, and large thunderclouds threaten to drench us.

> It seems to me, Olympe continues hurrying her pace, that there's a form of honesty in being able to say to your partner: 'I'm not going to dress up to look like a femme fatale, even if it's what gets you off, because it's simply not me.' But if I expect the other person

to accept me as I am, then I should be equally able to accept them as they are. Don't you think we should love each other for our true personalities, beyond these masculine or feminine stereotypes? Gender is a spectrum, and there are so many nuances! Let's have fun!

Let's have fun, I agree, not feeling entirely at ease.

Rome wasn't built in a day, Olympe says, smiling.

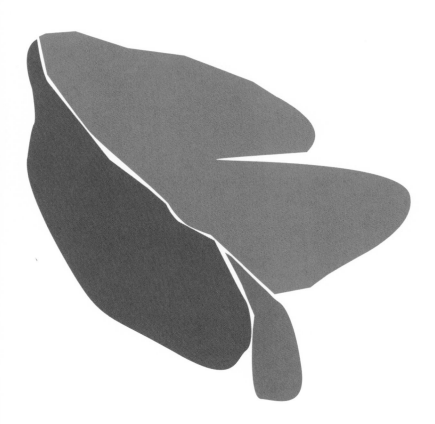

Going further

Odile Fillod, *a life-size clitoris for 3D-printing*

Odile Fillod is an independent researcher whose work sits at the crossroads of social science, biology and medicine. In 2016, noting that women all too often represent themselves with 'nothing' between their legs, she decided to create a 3D clitoris.[18] Basing her studies on up-to-date scientific literature, she devised the average size and shape of the clitoris. Her 3D model measures 10 centimetres, comprising the clitoral body with a right-angle bend at the glans, the two crura and the two bulbs attached under the main organ. Most importantly, it is available under a common creative licence, and can be printed out by anyone. Odile Fillod's work fights ignorance of the female anatomy – and, therefore, unequal access to pleasure between the sexes. Her work has had positive reverberations for learning among younger people: the way the clitoris is represented in French school textbooks has been improved.

Liv Strömquist, *The Origin of the World*

An extended essay in the form of a highly documented cartoon, *The Origin of the World* by Liv Strömquist[19] asks why female genital organs are considered shameful, incorrectly named and stigmatised. Rather than accepting the stock response, 'It's because we live in a patriarchal society,' she investigates those men (of the cloth, from the world of psychoanalysis, pedagogues, sexologists) who, over the centuries, have taken too great an interest in women's sexuality, to the point of transforming their obsession into full-blown campaigns of sexual repression. Did you know, for example, that Dr Kellogg, the inventor of cornflakes, was convinced that masturbation provoked womb cancer and epilepsy? He recommended burning the clitoris with acid! As for Dr Baker Brown, he recommended preventing women from pleasuring themselves by removing the clitoris (the last operation was carried out in 1948...). Periods, orgasms – Liv Strömquist shatters the misconceptions surrounding the vulva and the vagina.

Meg-John Barker and Jules Scheele, *Queer: A Graphic History*

An introduction to the history of queer thinking, this graphic novel[20] – more of an illustrated book than a cartoon – is both accessible and insightful. It invites the reader to ask themselves questions about gender and 'normality' alongside the founders of queer theory. How did Western culture find itself thinking that gender and sexuality are binary? And how does queer theory question this binary approach? The authors introduce some of the foremost thinkers – Alfred Kinsey, for example, who envisages sexuality as a spectrum, suggesting that people place themselves along a sliding scale and their position there is not fixed at all; or Judith Butler, for whom sexual behaviour is a performance, a role play that begins in childhood, along the lines of 'fake it until you make it'. This book takes all our preconceptions around gender identity, gender roles and what is 'normal' or 'natural' and turns them on their heads.

> How did Western culture find itself thinking that gender and sexuality are binary?

Michelle Ashford, *Masters of Sex*

Washington University, Saint-Louis, Missouri, 1956. Fertility expert Bill Masters launches an ambitious study on sexuality in a still markedly prudish America. Somewhat tongue-tied himself when it comes to discussing sex, he recruits Virginia Johnson, a brilliant young woman 100 per cent convinced that sex and loving feelings can be disassociated, and that sex can be enjoyed alone, without any need for sentimentality.

Based on Thomas Maier's eponymous biography of the two scientists, Bill Masters and Virginia Johnson, this series, developed by Michelle Ashford,[21] concentrates on fine-tuned aesthetic considerations and glamour (costumes, lights, etc.), and skilfully develops topics related to the research of Masters and Johnson: the place of women in a couple, the place of women in society, the moral judgements made about women who are not 'good mothers'. And another groundbreaking subject for the time: a woman's right to pleasure. As a single mother, Virginia Johnson is often torn between her career (for which she is frequently reproached) and her wish to spend time with her children. Johnson was the one responsible for the 'human science' side of the research, along with the university-based experiments. She recruited the volunteers who made love in the laboratory; she, too, was the one who listened to women – 'You can't quantify orgasms,' she stated – and allowed Johnson to refine his method of data collection.

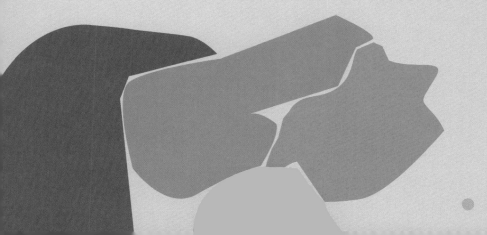

Annie Sprinkle, *How to be a Sex Goddess in 101 Easy Steps*

The Californian performer Annie Sprinkle is a pro-sex feminist icon. She believes that sex work and pornography can provide a means of re-appropriating one's body and sexuality. As an artist and activist, she has been promoting the teaching of a brand of whimsical and celebratory sex since the 1980s. In *How to be a Sex Goddess in 101 Easy Steps*,[22] she explores feminine pleasure with immense humour and wisdom at the same time. Seated against a green background that morphs into some very colourful images, Annie Sprinkle suggests we maximise our potential for orgasm by following her and her 'transformation facilitators' in this hour-long video guide.The journey begins with the rituals of preparation: beauty masks, wigs, make-up, outfits... But, take note, the ritual is not in any way limiting; on the contrary, it is deeply emancipating. The make-up can amount to face-painting; the hair-styling involves pubic hair; the outfits range from dominatrix to drag king, and also include cowgirl get-ups. And, if it's your thing, you can paint your body with menstrual blood.

Annie Sprinkle whispers to us that whoever we are, that person is welcome and deserves to be taken care of. Breathing exercises, dance and voice-warming exercises are appetisers to sexual pleasure. Behind the celebratory imagination of these 'goddesses' and 'sluts', Annie Sprinkle lays down the basics in this film: gender is a performance. Sexuality begins within. Every woman has different needs. Sex must be safe. Knowledge about female sexuality has been repressed, lost; it's time to re-appropriate it. And for us to get our orgasms back. It's a wonderful programme.

18 Odile Fillod's 3D-clitoris designs can be found at: https://www.thingiverse.com/thing:1876288.
19 Strömquist, L. 2016, *L'Origine de monde*, Rackham, Paris .
20 Barker, M. J. & Scheele, J. 2016, *Queer: A Graphic History*, Icon, London.
21 Ashford, M. 2013, *Masters of Sex*, Showtime.
22 Sprinkles, A. & Beatty, M. 1991, *The Sluts and Goddesses Video Workshop, or How to be a Sex Goddess in 101 Easy Steps*, Selfproduction.

Chapter 4

Understanding my needs and my limits

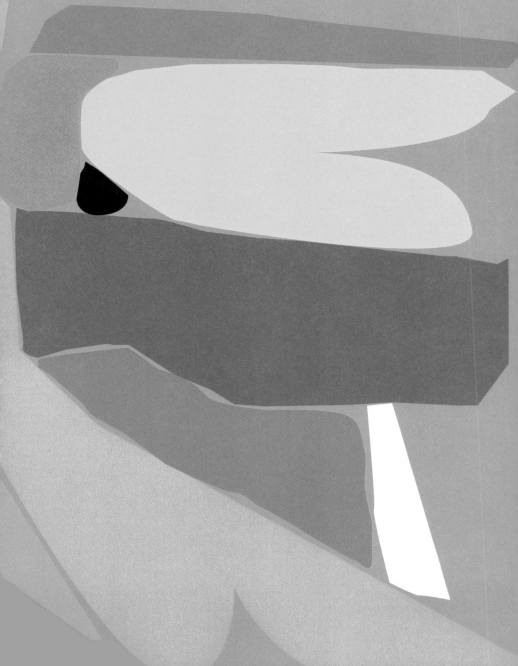

Thursday 19 August 2021

11.10am

Tomorrow, recording with Lélé for Voxxx.[23] Stéphanie will come to the recording, all the participants have given their consent to her presence which, I know, will be discreet and benevolent. Lélé and I have a number of texts on the agenda, including one that is a first for us, around the notion of 'invisible disability and pleasure'. A debut, too, for a new actor met last month – quite a high-pitched, breathy voice, who we hope will work his magic with the tens of thousands of listeners tuning in.

I would never have anticipated, when launching Voxxx in September 2018, that audio porn could be so successful. Having directed four sexually explicit short films (produced by Erika Lust) and acted in three,[24] I was keen to try something else. And then I had this audio experience, one totally unconnected to porn: wearing headphones I listened to a soundscape of being at the hairdresser's (as though I were in the chair, having my hair cut – *snip*, the scissors were close to my left ear, *snip*, at the back of my head). It gave me goosebumps from my head right down to my chest. After such a sensation, the idea took root: what about using not images but sounds to stimulate desire? If hairdressing scissors could bring on a shiver, imagine what would happen with sex scenes! What's more, we've all, at some time or other, in a hotel for instance, heard a couple losing themselves in their pleasure: if we don't know who they are and their voices are sexy, what could be more communicative?

That's how I came to be on a free porn site looking for voices to bring this audio-porn project to fruition. I wanted French-speaking, unique, personal and intimate voices. The problem is, porn tends to be very stereotypical, and its soundtracks are no exception – exaggerated moans that may even be out of sync with the action. And as for the dialogue – well, it's hmm... not exactly discerning. Finding voices that do it for me is anything but easy!

And then I came across Lélé O. Lélé is the queen of jerk-off instructions (JOI), a video genre that films a woman in front of the camera advising or directing the viewer about how to masturbate. Sound plays a fundamental role.

Lélé confounds the status quo, probably because she is at once sensitive and dominant, gentle and provocative. Thanks to clever framing, you don't see the upper half of her face. The focus is entirely on her mouth, on the words she chooses and slowly and indulgently utters. Her tone of voice is warm, serene. There is only one thing you want to do: follow her instructions and abandon yourself to your bliss.

Voxxx turned three this year. We've received a vast amount of enthusiastic feedback, some of it really touching, on our weekly audios. But what brought me most joy was imagining so many situations that you just don't *see* in classic porn. Situations that don't rush the performance, where it's all about taking the time to connect with your body. Situations involving different people, or those who experience their sensuality and sexuality differently. All with respect, joy and the constant reminder of what is meant by consent. During each recording, I feel like I'm prising open a door for an audience to bring them well-being and pleasure. And that is happiness!

7.25pm

Email from Stéphanie. She's sent me a link for the film *Chemistry Eases the Pain*, by Shine Louise Houston, which she's just come across on the website PinkLabel.tv. She's really enthusiastic about it. The film is a reflection on the internalised biphobia of the main character, Frankie. As a student, she is attracted to a guy in her chemistry class, Matt. But what should she do about her desire, having identified as a lesbian?

Aesthetically the film is beautiful and asks important questions. In addition, I realise it's been ages since I last watched any porn!

I discovered mainstream X-rated material aged nineteen, when I was going out with a guy ten years older than me. I worried about being sexually inadequate, about under-performing... I scoured free sites for what men fantasised about, how to give a blow job... I still remember my disbelief at the hundreds of videos alluding to incest. And the breasts, invariably enormous. Fast and furious thrusting groins, deep throat... It was all so far removed from me, from my body, from what I was able to do or bear. What I desired. I needed to take it slowly and gently. And when I switched off

63

my computer, I was even less sure of myself – and incapable of performing like that. I quickly decided to avoid that type of website.

8.45pm

Years later, aged thirty-three, I discovered feminist porn. What a revelation! I remember the thrill of watching a hooded activist, her pussy on show, masturbating in front of statues of 'great men' still celebrated despite the atrocities they wrought – for example, Christopher Columbus or Dr Sims. Through this film and many others, I discovered porn in the guise of protest and rebellion. There were also many videos filming feminine desire in a sensitive and realistic way: people grinding against pillows, lustfully whipping out their vibrators. I, at last, recognised my body and my desire in these films.

And I understood: that was what I wanted to do. To show women's sexualities and pleasure. To create representations of a partnership of equals. To produce beautiful pictures imbued with creativity and pride. To imagine that sex can provide a creative space.

Since starting my career work, I'd been able to produce some videos: I knew how to create images. So, I would strike out and direct a feminist porn film. But before standing behind the camera, it seemed important to be a performer myself. If I wanted to create proud images of the beauty of feminine sexuality, I couldn't do it hiding behind the camera lens! And how on earth could I imagine directing performers without knowing myself what it feels like to expose my own body?

I scroll through some photos on my screen. Click – me in suspenders, putting on make-up in front of a mirror; click – obscene graffiti; click – a long queue outside the KitKatClub. Click – an abandoned dome-shaped construction.

I shiver.

Immediately, I feel the sunshine of that Berlin afternoon when I'd been scouting for locations before shooting my first film, *The Bitchhiker*. The nearby wasteland. My good mood and all the hopes and ideas that bring my creative cooking pot to the boil.

My monkey spirit wants to drag me back to the difficulties I had during filming, the soul-searching I did at the time, my love life. Shut up, monkey spirit! *The Bitchhiker* is a beautiful film, and I'm proud of it. I love the shots where, clad in leather, I'm riding a motorbike early one morning; I love the very seventies feel, the psychedelic flares of pleasure. I love the idea that porn can be luminous and beautiful. How wonderful it would be if all women who want to put their sexuality on stage could do so! What a breath of freedom it would be for them!

9.25pm

Evening messages from my online community: 'I've just discovered Voxxx, it's beautiful, guilt-free – and how good it feels!'; 'You've got me to love porn, you've helped me feel at peace with love and tenderness, you've really helped me come into my own body, my desire and my sexuality'; 'I'm learning to listen to my body and my mind, I'm rediscovering myself.'

Well, I'd say my monkey spirit has taken itself off to bed!

9.50pm

Message from Stéphanie, who can't wait to attend to tomorrow's recording session. It's always amusing to look at our daily tasks from an outsider's point of view. Suddenly, what seemed nothing more than routine takes on a whole new dimension.

Stéphanie runs ctrlX,[25] an erotic podcast of recorded literary texts (Pierre Louÿs, John Cleland, Alina Reyes). ctrlX tells stories for adults – it's the narrative that counts. What's more, some of their audio creations, although they talk about sex, are not intended to arouse, but rather to amuse or lead to reflection. For example, there's a magnificent text from the 1960s by the Czech intellectual Jana Černá, *My Body Burns for your Mind*, that mingles love, basic desire, a refusal to submit oneself to a man, and a demand for individual freedom.

Sharing the audio recording experience with Stéphanie feels very natural. As though we both hail from the same distant country and have just met up there again. We've never discussed it, but I think we are similarly motivated in wanting to mix sex and audio.

Friday 27 August 2021

7.45am

Slept badly, too hot. Thank goodness the studio is air-conditioned!

10.10pm

What a day! I'm exhausted. Long recording session with Lélé. Actors coming and going. Intense concentration. One or two bouts of hysterical laughter that broke the tension. One incident (outside the studio) as well.

When I get there at 8am, Mélia, Voxxx sound engineer, is already in the process of preparing the session on the huge mixing console. Marc, the studio's sound engineer, places a microphone and stool in the recording room. We bring out clementines and hazelnut chocolate and drink coffee. It's the calm before the storm. In five minutes, the first voice will arrive, and then the second... And there'll be no stopping after that. Some of the performers are very experienced; others, making their first recordings, arrive in a state of excitement. Some of the episodes are easy to record – I know the performer well and they understand what I'm looking for. But it can be more complicated, take longer than expected. And so the tension mounts.

There is one thing that's especially difficult for me to manage in terms of direction: some professional actors have a 'melodic' voice that sounds like it should be in an ad or the dubbing for a TV series. It would be really insulting to tell someone whose voice is their professional tool that they sound like a French version of *Dallas*. I try to give a steer by offering prompts. When that falls through, it's just a matter of ingenuity. Whispering the episode, for example. Or perhaps interpreting the text as though they were on the cusp of orgasm all the way through. Acting out pleasure is an enormous challenge, even for theatre actors who are used to being on stage for hours at a time! It takes a lot of breath control, and it's not unusual for actors to hyperventilate and start seeing stars. Now we know, we watch out for it, but the first time an actor started becoming ill during a recording we weren't really prepared for it!

Stéphanie shuts her eyes when we start an episode in which there are only a few words and mainly sounds of contact, mouths and breathing. After ten minutes, she whispers in my ear:

Your skin tingles, then it reaches your groin. It's super arousing! And Lélé's voice is so warm. The effect is immediate. All you need do is close your eyes and you find your own mellow place.

I envy Stéphanie's ability to enjoy the hyper-immersive and personal aspects of these Voxxx episodes. Personally, I tend to focus on the dry-mouth 'clicking sounds' that require toning down, or pay attention to clumsy editing that will need fixing.

There's real intimacy in audio, says Stéphanie, and that's what makes it so powerful when you compare it to an image, isn't it? Each one of us can project what image we like based on what is being suggested. Just like when you read a book.

Yes! You can create your own porn film with your eyes shut. With the performers of your dreams... The sex positions you prefer... Your erotic imagination is a porn film in which everything is possible; that's what's so great about it. When writing, we try to avoid describing bodies as far as possible in Voxxx episodes, to give freedom to the listeners to picture them as they want.

It's obvious now you tell me, but I hadn't realised it before. Which just goes to show, it works!

You know how in old erotic novels, it's all about hairy chests, long, silky legs... We, on the other hand, can evoke a body without you guessing whether we're talking about a man or a woman. We allude to the chest, the nipples, the sex organs... Body parts that belong to all of us. And we also talk about becoming moist and getting a hard-on. Just like a clitoris becomes hard and a penis moist... All we know is that there is a body that's aroused. Each one of us can project what they want: a gender, a body shape, and so on. It means we can be as inclusive as possible.

I ask Stéphanie about her motivation for setting up ctrlX.

> I need stories, whether in my everyday reality or my sex life, all the time! she says. Porn no longer provides any.

> Except alternative X-rated porn! I remind her.

> That's true! You can still find storylines, and so much the better. When we set up ctrlX, the idea was to be carried away by a storyline. You're told a beautiful sex tale, penned by a talented writer. Sure, of course, it's not as 'powerful' as Voxxx. But you see what I'm getting at.

She smiles:

> That's another way of doing it. But with the same idea of having a good time with yourself with a focus on pleasure.

A round of lemonade

We record two texts without much difficulty. The third turns out to be more complicated. The performer hasn't slept because of the heat. His voice is therefore even deeper than usual, and that's great. However, he forces his words, gets frustrated, and the overall effect is unnatural, lacking flow and desire. Lélé, feeling the tension rise on both sides of the studio window, suggests we have a break, and Stéphanie and I leave the building to get a breath of fresh air. The sun has not yet reached its zenith, and we sit on a shady terrace to enjoy some lemonade.

> Do you think audio porn is the ethical future of pornography, asks Stéphanie, twirling bits of lemon pulp with her paper straw.

> Audio or film... We should be able to offer really good pornography in any format. I love Voxxx, but if I could get the funding, I'd really like to make another film. I'd choose performers I want to work with, and I'd be able to pay them properly, including for rehearsals.

I'd have cameras and lenses that would allow me to realise my creative goals. I could, for a change, pay all the team members properly for their commitment and expertise. The problem is, there's no money for sexually explicit films.

Everyone looks at pornography, but no one is prepared to pay to view it!

That's just it! Society has got used to accessing it for free, and production companies don't believe the genre is real cinema.

You have to admit that what you can watch on free streaming platforms isn't...

I agree.

They're videos made on a shoestring and working conditions are often appalling, I say. Poor treatment on X-rated movie sets makes people more indignant than was previously the case, but it's still a topic that people prefer to sweep under the carpet. 'After all, individuals *choose* to star in X-rated films; if they're badly treated, they've only got themselves to blame': that's what most people believe. It's a line of argument used for sex workers in general.

My first porn film

Out of the corner of my eye, I notice a sideways glance from a woman sitting at the next table. She might be thirty-something, busy on her laptop. She's removed her headphones and keeps turning her head in our direction – perhaps because of my tattoos). More likely because of what we're discussing. I carry on.

If I have decided to be filmed having sex, it's because I was convinced I shouldn't be ashamed of my body or my sexuality. I want women to be proud of their desires and their pleasure.

That was my message and the battle I was waging.

Porn, for you, has been a way of growing into yourself as a woman, replies Stéphanie. Of accepting yourself, loving yourself and re-appropriating your body. But that's your experience. What I'm saying is that we can't all be porn stars – we don't all have that relationship with our own intimacy.

In my relations with men, I already enjoyed performing: taking photos and filming myself. And, yes, I'm well aware that not all women want to undress in front of a camera lens.

Aren't you afraid you'll lose control of these videos? It's no small thing to have intimate videos at large in the big wide world...

I nod in agreement.

It should be said over and again that any photo or video that is shared is then completely out of your control, I say. Personally, I've been had. All my films have been pirated and made available on free platforms – without permission, of course. While I was happy with the idea of showing my body and expressing my pleasure to a feminist audience, I had no intention whatsoever of exposing myself on a free streaming platform with a vast audience – you find private videos on these same sites, ones that have only been sent to one individual.

Yes, revenge porn... It's become a massive phenomenon and it's very worrying, like those slut-shaming, fisha accounts. Do you still send nude pictures?

Well, yes! I laugh. It gives me a real kick to pose, to be desired. And in addition, I want to believe that you can still trust people, even on a straightforward date. That there isn't a wolf always lurking on the net. Don't you send any?

Our neighbour at the next table gathers up her belongings.

I'm sorry to butt in, she says, without looking directly at us (initially, I wonder if she's even talking to us). What you're saying is shocking. Perhaps when you're a professional like yourself there are no taboos, but that's not the case for everyone. And I can't stay silent when I hear you saying that pornography can be good for women.

A teaspoon falls to the ground with a sharp clang; the woman doesn't bother picking it up. She rummages furiously in her bag.

No worries, Stéphanie says gently. I'm sorry if our conversation upset you. We should have been more careful.

I'm a feminist, continues the woman, still angry. And to be honest, I'm shocked. Porn is something for guys, where they learn how to dominate us in bed. It's a tool of the patriarchy to make us objects of 'their' pleasure.

A tool. Well it depends what use you make of it, I hear myself answering.

Don't feed the troll

Stéphanie shoots a look in my direction as if to say, *OK, let's allow the storm to pass.* But there is always a small voice inside that wants to believe that dialogue is possible.

Stéphanie's right, I say. Sorry if we've shocked you; it wasn't our intention. Allow me just to say one thing: I thought like you do, until the day I discovered there are other types of porn to the kind you see everywhere, the kind created by heterosexual men for heterosexual men. There are respectful portrayals, created while ensuring full consent from the performers, and that focus on female pleasure. *Real* female pleasure, involving the clitoris, care and sensitivity, maybe using lube... It's this type of pornography – the feminist type – that I'm talking about. If I defend it, it's because

it has helped me take possession of my body, of my pleasure.
If we have more women directors, then the whole way we look
at sex changes. Do you see what I mean?

Our interlocutor scowls. She's put her bag on the table and no longer
appears to be on the defensive.

Because you really think you can stand up to all those productions
that flood the web and treat us like meat? she demands. Those films
put women in danger. And you'll never stop me believing that this
so-called empowerment of a female sex worker over her body
is anything other than a crude ploy on the part of the patriarchy.
You see yourself as a liberated woman because you make
pornography. I think you're talking crap.

Stéphanie tucks a banknote under the carafe and stands up.

They're waiting for us, she tells me.

I seize the opportunity and follow her out. It's only later that
we discuss the morning incident further.

I just don't understand these people who ram their beliefs
down your throat, groans Stéphanie. If you like making porn,
what on earth has it got to do with anyone else?

That's exactly the point: it's about stepping out of your box and
understanding that the choices you could never make might be
fulfilling for someone else. And that goes for sexuality as a whole.
I encourage everyone to know themselves and take possession
of whatever they genuinely enjoy – I don't say you must do this
or that. It's up to the individual to explore, make their choices
and weigh the risks.

Stéphanie gives a nod.

The same is true for sexual practices, she says. Maybe anal sex suits one person but not another. That doesn't mean there has to be a scale of values.

To seek what's good for you, without putting yourself in danger: I think that's the fundamental point.

Sunday 5 September 2021

6.45pm

Message from Stéphanie about her relationship to porn: 'X-rated material was an education. I watched it, I stopped watching when I didn't enjoy it – I'm saying this because sometimes I get the impression people feel duty-bound to watch things simply because they've started.

Porn made me want to try a range of experiences. Some of these quickly disappeared from my imagination. Others took over as enduring fantasies. A few needed putting to the test – opened up avenues that were appealing.'

The educational side of pornography is a complex issue. And that's without even mentioning the fact that children see images *that they should not see* – adolescents and young adults are able to view all sorts of practices on free X-rated websites, in the absence of any context, deconstruction or explanation. I think pornography *shouldn't* be available to watch for free. But as it is, because that's the reality, our teenagers, in their secondary and high schools, should be guided through it.

Today, in France, information about sex and sex education is compulsory during primary and secondary education, and pupils are given at least three classes on them per year. It's not much – and worse still, these sessions practically do not take place. We keep telling ourselves that because pupils have been learning about 'sexual reproduction in living beings' or contraception, or risks of STDs, sexuality is acknowledged. But does the same go for consent, sexual violence, gender identity, the existence of variations in genital development, sexual orientation, respect and the relationship with one's body and one's pleasure? Porn will never replace words, exchanging information, education. All the studies that have been conducted on the impact of a comprehensive sex education on children show that teaching them about anatomy, physiology, tolerance, inclusion, gender, consent, body image, communication ... leads to less sexual assault, fewer STIs, fewer unwanted pregnancies and later age of first intercourse. Offering an educational approach to sexuality that is both positive and respectful does not make teens want to engage in a shared sexual life earlier; it makes them want to engage in sexuality better!

I receive messages from girls, still in their teens, on my Voxxx Instagram account. They tell me they're pleased to have discovered safe erotic content. They're scared about coming across images that they won't be able to forget if they go on to porn sites. I would love to be able to point them in the direction of purely educational content. Why are there no videos or podcasts that can answer these adolescents' questions?

Instagram accounts play a role in sex education and in deconstructing trash porn. But it seems appropriate that this task should primarily fall to educators who are specifically trained in these issues.

It is important to tell everyone that fiction can arouse us, inspire us, but isn't reality. It's the reflection of a certain vision of the world, an approach to our person-to-person relationships. If Pornhub or X-Hamster tell us *ad nauseam* that heterosexual sex ends in ejaculation over the face, not only is that a lie, it's also a way of promoting sexual behaviour centred on masculine domination. In real life, as the song goes, 'Do what you please.'

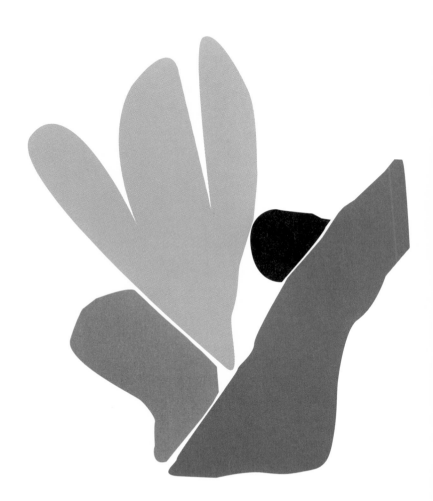

23 Voxxx (www.voxxx.org): an audio platform offering guided, immersive, inclusive and intimate masturbation sessions.
24 As a performer: *Un beau dimanche*, by Lucie Blush, 2016; *The Bitchhiker*, by Olympe de Gê., 2016; *Architecture Porn*, by Erika Lust, 2017. As a director: *The Bitchhiker*, 2016; *Don't Call Me a Dick*, 2017; *Take Me Through the Looking Glass*, 2017; *We are the Fucking World*, 2017.
25 *ctrlX*, ctrlX.fr: erotic and pornographic readings in new sound settings…

Buck Angel

'What it means
to be a man or
a woman depends
100 per cent
on the individual'

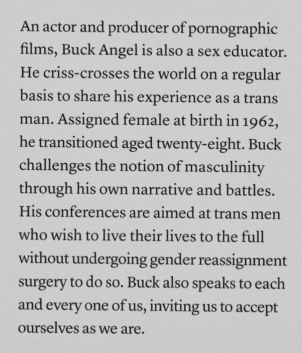

An actor and producer of pornographic films, Buck Angel is also a sex educator. He criss-crosses the world on a regular basis to share his experience as a trans man. Assigned female at birth in 1962, he transitioned aged twenty-eight. Buck challenges the notion of masculinity through his own narrative and battles. His conferences are aimed at trans men who wish to live their lives to the full without undergoing gender reassignment surgery to do so. Buck also speaks to each and every one of us, inviting us to accept ourselves as we are.

Stéphanie Estournet (SE)   What does it mean to be a man or a woman? Is there a definition we can provide, or is it up to each of us to give our own definition?

Buck Angel (BA)   If we talk about what we feel and not specifically about biological facts, defining what it is to be a man or a woman depends 100 per cent on the individual. For me, the thing that defines me as a man is the way I feel, how I interact with the world, how people see me.

My level of confidence increased significantly after my physical transition to appear masculine. Before transitioning, I looked much more feminine, somewhat androgynous; people sometimes couldn't work out whether I was a woman or a man. It was very important for me to be seen as a man. Since being able to live my life without anyone mistaking my identity, my self-confidence has rocketed.

SE   I guess you have had to work hard on yourself to understand who you are...

BA   Actually, I've known who I am for a long time. At school, I used to say, 'I feel I'm a boy.' I was told, 'Shut up, you're just a tomboy; it's fine, you'll get over it.'

Olympe de Gê   And you didn't listen to them. You had to carve out your own path to travel the world as a man.

BA   Believe me, it hasn't always been easy. I have no idea how others manage to gain confidence in who they are. In my case, it took me a long time to get there and understand I didn't need validation. In reality, we live in a world where everything – especially what we are – seems to be linked to validation from others. Look at how we behave on social media – even me, you know! We're looking for validation from likes, from interaction with people who will – genuinely – help us become more confident through telling us how great we are. But as soon as everything depends on comments from people you don't know, this feeling of security and confidence is worthless.

SE   When you acted in porn films, did you ask yourself about pushing the boundaries?

BA   When I started acting in X-rated films, my main motivation was to earn money. Lots of money. I wanted to do business. Trans men were not being portrayed in pornography at all. Only trans women. To be honest with you, during those first films I didn't realise what we were doing was so powerful.

O de G   You mean you didn't intend to stray into political or educational issues?

BA   Exactly. I did it in order to earn my living. Also because there was a creative side to the work. But at the end of the day, it didn't turn out as I had hoped (laughter). Porn isn't really the place to make a fortune, except for the odd exception!

O de G   But you carried on...

BA   I gradually understood that I was pushing the boundaries with my pornography: I was the man with the vagina. For the first time, these identity questions were reaching a wider audience. And I was the one making it possible, at last, to be able to push the boundaries. I realised the impact of my films, and from that moment on, I started taking part in conferences around the world.

SE   Do you encourage people to consume pornography?

BA   I encourage people to look at porn, definitely! But I'm always careful to warn people. I am convinced that pornography doesn't suit everyone. It's important for each of us to understand that you can be distressed or maybe disturbed by something you watch in porn scenes. Pornography is everywhere, but that's not a reason to trivialise it. But I still have great faith in using pornography as an educational tool.

O de G   Should educational environments (schools, educators, and so on) play a role in helping people accept themselves and in sex education, or are these private issues that should be discussed at home, in the family or with a therapist?

BA   It's a difficult question to answer. One thing is certain: communicating positive values about bodies and their differences seems, to me, to be really important.

SE   You can nevertheless understand the warnings about swapping 'homemade' pornographic films.

BA   That's true. Today, many young people don't understand what it means to be naked on the internet, how vulnerable it makes us. The fact is that in the majority of cases, you can't remove photos or films even if you want to. We need to be educated about these issues and understand the potential repercussions and risks.

O de G   What can we learn from pornography? Can it play a positive role in sex education for young adults?

BA   We can learn so many things! Love for oneself, the beauty of other types of bodies, other types of people, other ways to make love. Pornography has enabled me to connect to my own body and my own pleasure. That's how I learned to masturbate, and discovered how powerful some sex toys can be. Pornography is still very controversial, but I'm convinced it's an important vector for sex education. I hope we will keep on changing our outlook and can approach it in future as a tool for finding our pleasure.

Going further

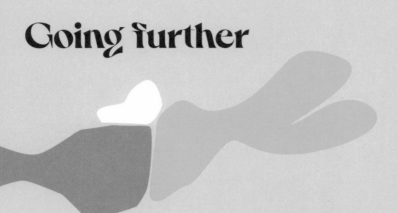

Skyler Braeden Fox, *The 36-year-old Virgin*

Performer and producer Skyler, a trans man aged thirty-six, wishes to feel what it's like to have penetrative sex for the first time with a cis-man. Basically, he'd like to have a 'traditional' penis-vagina intercourse. When D-Day arrives, Skyler chooses to have this experience with Bishop Black. However, from his imagination to the actual deed, there is a world of emotions, and, at the final moment, a mental block! Skyler won't, in the end, film the expected footage, and that's what is so precious: watching a porn film that doesn't film what it was supposed to film... and stops partway through to ask questions.

Olympe de Gê, *Don't Call Me a Dick*

'Dick, arsehole, prick'... Why are these words insults when they derive from body parts that are so good for us? Olympe made this short film in 2017 for the Erika Lust platform. It was shot in macro and very slowed down, thereby injecting poetry and emotion into the close-ups of genitals that are so common in mainstream porn. The spectacular images (including a squirt at 1,000 images a second!) offer a different view of the beauty of sex in general, and of genitals in particular.

Jim and Artie Mitchell, *Behind the Green Door*

This film needs to be viewed in its context: the 1970s. In many ways, it doesn't reflect what one would expect of a progressive porn film today: the heroine is kidnapped (bingo, rape culture); the main actor's Black body is fetichised (tribal collar, cut-off long johns that seem to reduce the personage to his penis). Nonetheless, let's be humble: there is every chance that in fifty years' time, people will quake when looking at the images that we are creating as best we can today. So let's pay homage to this film, despite its irritating premise, and enjoy its extraordinary visual inventiveness. The images attempt to express sexual pleasure in an innovative way, moving away from the clichéd close-ups of contorted faces, fingers clutching at the sheets, etc... It reminds one a little of Ingmar Bergman with the flattened effect of its strong colours, before it shifts into experimentation, terminating in a completely psychedelic scene of final ejaculations.

Ovidie, *Pornocratie*

Why is that porn is going through an immense expansion on the internet (where it takes up about 30 per cent of available bandwidth!), while at the same time production conditions for X-rated movies have collapsed and actors are the prime victims? In this documentary, Ovidie investigates why porn performers end up filming scenes that are twice as 'hard' but for half the money. It illustrates how this major upheaval in the X-rated film industry is linked to the arrival of online video-sharing platforms (*YouPorn*, *Pornhub*, *Xhamster*, etc.). Set up by geeks to make a quick buck, these platforms put up free videos that can be viewed an unlimited number of times, most of which are bootlegs, and it's total anarchy. *Pornocratie* strongly emphasises that consuming free porn because 'it doesn't cost anything' and 'everyone does it' leads to propping up an unfair and abusive system. #payforyourporn.

81

Chapter 5

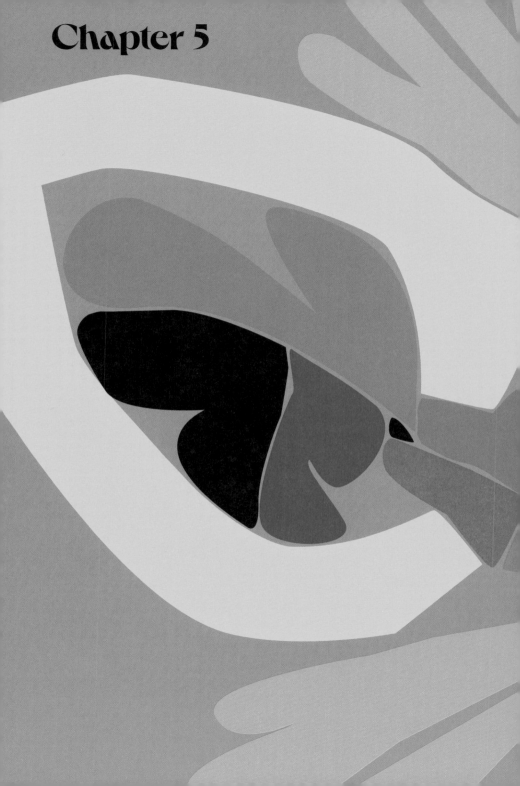

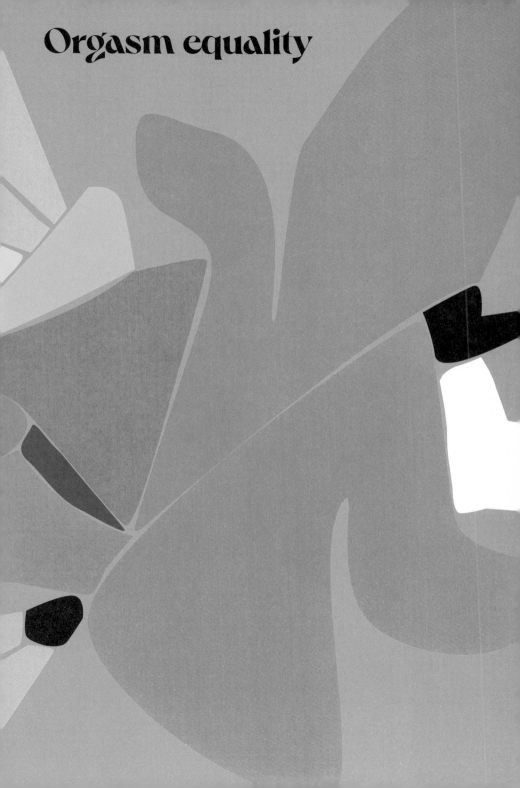

Orgasm equality

Today's meeting place is the Cirque Electrique: a friendly space with an old-fashioned big top on the edge of Paris. People come to dance, have a drink and, of course, to see shows. I suggested the place to Olympe. Otomo De Manuel, a performer I've been following as a journalist for several years, is rehearsing his *Le Cabaret Décadent* show with a troupe of performers.[26] *Le Cabaret Décadent* offers the customary circus routines – juggling, acrobatics and trapeze acts – but in punk and queer mode.

> Central to this show, Otomo explains, is the anger we harbour
> against cowardice and convention, against narrow thought
> processes. There is also a hunger to beat stupidity through
> laughter, and to do exactly what we want with our bodies
> by being who we are.

Olympe is certainly enjoying my choice of venue. I can see it in her faint smile – and in the increasingly intrigued look in her eyes as the performers file in. With his tattooed, athletic body and luscious lips, pouting insolently and throwing us a sultry look, the pole dancer, Quentin Dée, enters the ring. He's joined by another athletic body, the aerial acrobat and contortionist Julie Demont.

> These artists are extraordinarily beautiful, whispers Olympe
> as we settle ourselves in the stands.

> Otomo flashes his cockchafer-gold fingernails as he points
> to the catering bar.

> I have to leave you, he says. I'll be back in a while. Help yourselves
> to a drink or whatever else you would like, OK?

Otomo rejoins the circus performers in the centre of the ring. Some are sitting on chairs taken from the spectators' area, others are juggling, stretching their muscles. People are smoking cigs and drinking coffee. There is something gleefully improper in their attitudes.

Otomo had briefed me: the troupe holds a pre-rehearsal meeting to debrief the previous day's show and sort out any day-to-day matters.

I wanted to observe this moment with Olympe to gauge the atmosphere. It's for moments like these that I love live performance. It doesn't matter how well-known the show or the troupe is: when you get the opportunity to be invited to a workplace meeting or a rehearsal, it's as though you were suddenly being allowed into the kitchens of a gourmet restaurant. Each person appears exactly as they are and as they feel. And the troupe is there, in all its individual variety and strength. What's more, *Le Cabaret Décadent*'s company is special in questioning the limits of gender and has several genderfuck performers, as Otomo likes to call them. Each artiste is themself in their own way – and their brazenness is exhilarating for the audience.

It's cool being here, but I can't really find any direct link to today's subject, says Olympe, sweeping her eyes over the performers.

It's true that for today, we had set out to tackle the place of women in heterosexual relationships. To explain my choice, I could mention my joy at seeing Otomo, with his long-legged, gangly gait, alpha-male signalling while dressed in a corset, fishnet tights and stilettos. Or else I could talk about how I feel somehow in disguise when I put on a suspender belt or a pair of stilettos, although I feel 100 per cent woman. I could share my astonishment at the roles straight women and straight men play without even realising it. But instead, I choose to re-contextualize our subject:

Women's pleasure is almost always a secondary event in straight intercourse – as if the woman were destined to excite the man, who is allowed to enjoy his pleasure as much as he wants.

Olympe interrupts me:

Wait, that's a bit pessimistic! There are men who very actively seek the pleasure of women ...

I look at her with surprise. She continues:

...to better inflate their ego, and reassure themselves on their virility!

We laugh. I get back to my train of thoughts:

Seriously, though... Why don't we break free from this role
we've been assigned? Why not – like Otomo, Julie, Quentin and
the others – choose how we want to be rather than behave
as is expected of us, even in our intimate lives?

Otomo chooses this precise moment move into the middle of the ring, rolling his hips in his super-high heels. He announces in his deep voice:

Ladies and gentlemen, bitches, freaks and queers...
Olympe has been thinking.

Reject our role as second fiddle in bed... she murmurs.
OK, I follow your train of thought.

And choose to take control of our own pleasure. No longer being
the woman who bottles up her frustrations because that's 'just how
it is'; the woman who is used to not being heard when she says
penetration hurts; who is reluctant to admit she can't get an orgasm
with men; who loves deep kisses, but struggles to say that she
would prefer not to have her vulva touched. The woman who,
having faked it so often, can no longer behave otherwise...

Olympe smiles.

That reminds me of the beginning of *King Kong Theory*:[27]
'I write from the realms of the ugly, for the ugly, older women,
women lorry drivers, the frigid, the unfucked and the unfuckable,
the drama queens, the crazies, all those excluded from the great
meat market of female flesh,' she quotes.

Why shouldn't I climax as often as you do?

According to an American study from 2017,[28] 95 per cent of heterosexual men have an orgasm during shared sexual activity. The percentage of heterosexual women in this category is only 65 per cent. A 2019 study indicated that two thirds of French women had, at some time, faked an orgasm – a percentage that has almost doubled in twenty years (from 32 per cent in 1998 to sixty-two in 2019). This orgasm gap is, in itself, a marker of an inequality between men and women that permeates down to our sexuality.

> *Especially* with regards to our sexuality, Olympe corrects. And to all those men and women who would like to believe that there is a biological explanation for the fact that a man can orgasm more easily – because his penis is external – I would like to remind them of this: 86 per cent of lesbian women always or almost always reach orgasm during shared sexual activity.

> While the difference between straight and gay men is almost insignificant.

> So the problem isn't the women, but the place they are expected to occupy in the relationship. I am also convinced that the predominance of the penis in heterosexual relationships, the way it is at the centre of everything, creates an imbalance in the relationship from the outset.

In the ring, Quentin Dée is warming up, dressed in shorts, his bare, tattooed chest glistening with sweat.

> I always feel somewhat embarrassed criticising the penis as the origin of all our woes, I admit. After all, if I want an orgasm, I know how to get one, whether during a shared sexual experience or alone.

> But do you? asks Olympe, smiling. I mean, you know what I'm getting at: there are so many women, especially young women, who don't dare touch themselves while they're having sex. Because

it's not the done thing, because we've been told that it's a childish, immature way of pleasuring ourselves, because we are supposed to love 'cock'... and not our fingers. Man can climax to the point of drunkenness, hump away, wank off. Women, on the other hand, must stick to their role – to excite – but they mustn't imagine their pleasure in a selfish manner. That would be obscene, unacceptable.

I am well aware of this internalised restraint that we all have, to some degree or other. At the same time, I feel we could just place our hands on our clitorises, or elsewhere, and not give a fig about being watched by our partner. Even to open his eyes to the fact that we are giving ourselves the pleasure he can't necessarily provide.

Some women can do that, Olympe qualifies. Unfortunately, from the moment that we accept our roles without much further thought, a large number of us are unable to find the courage to take our pleasure in hand – if I can put it that way. Perhaps to some extent because our partner might take it badly that we can bring ourselves to orgasm while he doesn't manage to give us this pleasure.

I shake my head.

If I want to touch myself, whether I'm alone or with someone, I do it, don't I? I say. Being watched by a man shouldn't be seen as validating or invalidating my actions.

Olympe takes a moment to find the right words.

I totally agree, she says eventually. But for me, this stance leads to another question: where is equality if we are able to make men orgasm using our mouths, our hands, and by rubbing them

86 per cent of lesbian women always or almost always reach orgasm during shared sexual activity.

with our bodies, while they are often incapable of doing the same for us? Of course, I could use my favourite toy during sex, and I'm completely in favour of having shared moments of masturbation.

To look and be looked at...

But for the sake of equality, would it not be necessary for men to pleasure us just like we can pleasure them?

Practical work and assessments

A circus babe comes into the ring, swathed in white feathers, twirling to the sound of a Nino Rota-style tune.

Olympe makes a good point. Used as I am to looking after my partners, and *delighted* as I am when they (genuinely) look after me, I had never considered the relationship to the female orgasm in this way. What would it mean to be – truly – on equal terms when it comes to pleasure? I get excited:

That would mean they would have to learn...

Long-term training...

With practical assignments and end-of-term assessments!

Olympe and I laugh, but this notion of training suddenly seems serious and fundamental. I understood early on that I couldn't count on my male partners to bring me to orgasm. In any case, I remember not expecting anything from them, right from my first sexual experiences. It's pretty sad when you think about it. Such an attitude implies that I had internalised – unconsciously, of course – the fact that, for my own pleasure I could only count on myself. If a partner showed himself to be interested in genuine sharing, I felt I'd hit the jackpot. But I had no expectations after he exited the scene – nah, nah, nah.

Today, in the light of Olympe's suggestion, I ask myself whether we shouldn't seriously consider our jokey suggestion about ultimately training straight men about women's orgasms. For my part, I have chosen to adopt the following attitude: I will no longer fake or play at total fulfilment when I'm not feeling it (without being unpleasant about it, an orgasm – whether his or hers – isn't a given). Instead, I propose guiding his caresses, and, if we feel comfortable talking about it, discussing our preferences to make clear what we each enjoy and find less enjoyable (no, our groans are not enough). This might be something that we explore together in the heat of the action, but equally, it might be worth pointing him in the direction of texts and Instagram accounts that we've found really excellent on this subject.[29]

The trumpet tune has finished. The babe dons a white-feather headdress and discusses something with the musician.

To our knowledge, no long-term, intensive training programme exists that could turn our partners into Graduates of Clitoral Studies, specialising in erogenous zones. On reflection, that might not necessarily be such a good thing. Although some would be awarded degrees, even first-class honours, others would fail.

It can't all be down to us yet again, notes Olympe.

Not everything, no. But neither can we cross our arms and wait until something happens, on the pretext that the ball's in their court. It's a game for two: men and women. Don't you agree?

Pink fur or cunnilingus: what does it for you?

The babe has disappeared and it's Pierre Pleven and Quentin Dée's turn. Both clad in shorts and heels, they throw themselves into their pole-dance routine.

All good with you girls? asks Otomo, grabbing a chair to join us. He turns the chair seat towards him and settles on to it, cowboy-style, leaning his arms on the back. Was there something in particular you wanted to talk about? he asks.

I nod.

For us, the idea is to tear down the secondary role of the woman in heterosexuality, I explain. Rather like *Le Cabaret Décadent* subverts gender stereotypes. I was thinking that, with your experience, you'd have some suggestions. I imagine you've had to fight against dos and don'ts to be the person you are today, haven't you?

Otomo lights up a cigarette and offers us the packet.

The similarity I can see between my experience and your subject is the idea of taking hold of yourself, he says. And deconstructing yourself. He exhales a puff of smoke, then continues: Look at my body shape – I'm tall. And because I'm tall, I ought to have taken up basketball. Because I come from a military family, I ought to have joined the armed services. That's how all this began. As a little boy, I deconstructed all those things that didn't suit me, all the pigeon holes people kept putting me in. He pauses. Gazing reflectively into the middle distance, he goes on: Of course, the moment came when I either had to shut up or react. And after that, things followed a similar pattern. I wanted to dress like a girl. And so what? If I decide to wear a dress, I know I'm going to have to defend myself against idiots stuck in their knee-jerk reactions. But what's the alternative? Giving up what I am? What suits me?

Olympe smiles.

I don't know many men able to say to themselves: I want to wear heels or a skirt... she says.

Otomo gestures with his arm toward the ring.

There are some like that right there, he says. Pierre Pleven, for example. Pierre explains bloody fantastically about being considered gay because he likes dancing and wearing heels. He was unhappy at being thought gay when he wasn't. He stopped everything. And then an opportunity arose, and he slipped back into his stilettos and dancing.

I smile.

An accessory can't define your sexuality, I say.

More broadly, we have to stop limiting ourselves, reducing things down to stereotypes, Otomo says. That goes for our looks; and for our sexuality. We need to keep saying, over and over again: the first thing is to understand who you are. Spend some time asking yourself if you like this or that. If this or that experience was enjoyable. There is also a moment when we have to question what has been stuffed into our heads simply because we are a guy or a girl. That way, we can deconstruct it all if it doesn't suit us. When we know who we really are, deep down, we are in a position to defend our tastes, our choices, what suits us, on a different level from the diktats imposed on men and on women.

From the sound booth, someone is calling Otomo's name, and he waves to signal he's on his way.

You can sometimes feel comfortable in a pigeon hole, but, in truth, your wings are clipped, he continues. Sexually, if you question yourself and alter your viewpoint from time to time, it allows you to ask yourself questions: do I feel like doing this or that? You learn to know yourself, to trust in yourself. From that point onwards, you are more spontaneous and move towards what's good for you rather than what we're told is good for us – you get my drift? He tosses his pink furry jacket over his shoulders and replaces the chair. Girls, he says, I have to dash, we've still got things to sort out in the sound booth. You'll come and watch the show?

Of course we'll come to see the show. If only to applaud these talents whose overt deconstruction provides a light at the end of the patriarchal tunnel.

In an ideal world

Seated on a terrace further down the hill from the circus, Olympe and I enjoy the shade of the parasols, the chaises longues and iced citrus fruit juice.

These guys and girls are fabulous, and they all look so strong, notes Olympe. I guess that's normal when you are using your muscles and keeping your balance all day.

And risking your life on a trapeze bar or walking a tightrope. They do look strong, I agree. And also – how can I put it? – so anchored to the ground. As though nothing, outside their personal choices, could knock them.

Olympe takes off her sunglasses and looks at me.

In my ideal world, she says, I would be like them in my sexual relationships: at ease, doing what I want with my body – with or without body hair, curvy or slim, salt and pepper or dyed hair, or even shaven-headed. I would feel sexy because I would be living in the moment, giving in to my impulses. I would feel sexy because of the bond between my partner and myself – not because I'd put on suspenders to make my new date happy.

I seize the image and respond in kind.

In my ideal world, it's not just me being penetrated. I say. My partner doesn't have the usual inhibitions about penetration, andhas discovered he enjoys being penetrated. And we just go with the flow, penetrate each other if we feel like it. Or not. We fall silent while the waiter refills our glasses.

In my ideal world, Olympe continues, pornography shows women taking the initiative, climaxing, freely and beautifully, while their partner looks on – things don't come to an end once the man has ejaculated.

In my ideal world, we don't talk about foreplay any more. There are no rules about the order in which things happen, or pre-set ways of doing things. Penetration as the main dish has been taken off the menu, because penetrating and being penetrated are just some among an array of pleasures. We suck our ice cubes, giggling like adolescents.

Our world's going to be great, says Olympe with a smile.

I cringe.

We've got a long way to go before we get there ... I say.

26 Created and staged by Hervé Vallée.
27 Despentes, V. 2010, *King Kong Theory*, Feminist Press, New York – the book was presented by her editor, Grasset, as 'a pamphlet for a new feminism'.
28 Frederick, D. A., John, H. K. S., Garcia, J. R. *et al.* February 2017, 'Differences in Orgasm Frequency Among Gay, Lesbian, Bisexual and Heterosexual Men and Women in a U.S. National Sample,' *Archives of Sexual Behaviour*, vol. 47, no. 1, pp. 273–288.
29 It seems vital to mention Jüne Plã's *Bliss Club* (Hardie Grant, 2020), a hands-on sex-education manual that explains, through illustrations and in simple language, how to give your partner pleasure, whatever their gender.

Martin Page

'Some types of oppression need to be eradicated from, what on the surface, seems natural and obvious'

French fiction writer Martin Page also writes as an essayist on societal topics. Published in 2019, his book *Beyond Penetration* raises the possibility of heterosexual relations no longer being centred on penetration, but leaving room for other experiences (stroking, kissing, etc.) – and for heightened pleasure for women.

Olympe de Gê (O de G)   Where did the idea for your book come from, considering you say in your essay that you 'love the act of penetration'?

Martin Page (MP)   As often happens when I throw myself into an essay – it's especially true when I write about vegetarianism – the topic plays a major role in my daily life. So, while talking to girlfriends of mine, I made a shocking discovery: many women don't feel satisfied by traditional heterosexual sex involving penetration. Yet they put up with it, because it's the norm. They force themselves. It's what's expected of them. And, what's more, they don't want to disappoint their partners. These discussions led me to reconsider my views on sexuality in general, but also on a personal level. I like penetration, but I believe it's important, when in a dominant position, to criticise what one likes. Some types of oppression need to be eradicated from what, on the surface, seems natural and obvious.

Stéphanie Estournet (SE)   How have the men around you reacted to your research?

MP   Men don't discuss sex much. When they do talk about it, it's often in terms of achievement; they are marking their position on the macho scale by comparing the number of women they've slept with. They are devoid of any sense of self-reflection. If they're not show-offs, then it's their shyness that comes to the fore. Basically, they talk about sex poorly, or not at all.

In my book, I wanted to engage with men because of their inability to find the right words. But I realise I missed my target: 95 per cent of those who buy my book are women!

O de G   Which confirms, if proof were needed, that women read and find things out.

MP   Yes, they're curious about change. That's less true of men because they are the dominant ones and so don't need (or want) to educate themselves or change.

SE   Your premise is that penetration is a given in straight sex – the man penetrating the woman, of course. The majority of women only feel moderate pleasure with this: the man, on the contrary, climaxes most of the time. And yet straight sex is still the norm…

MP   Originally, penetration was, of course, tied up with our instinct to reproduce. With the arrival of contraception, pleasure has taken centre stage in our sexual relationships. But penetration still remains the benchmark of 'proper' heterosexual sex that satisfies men, but far less often satisfies women.

   In an ideal world, we would ask ourselves: 'Right, what are we going to do to move towards more equality in our pleasure?' We're far from that right now. If it's still a difficult topic to bring up – in society at large, within couples, or even with yourself – it's because it uncovers a reality that goes beyond the scope of sex: the domination of one social group over another.

O de G   Right into one's intimate sphere…

MP   In 2012, exactly ten years ago, *ELLE* magazine advocated blow jobs as 'what cements a couple together'. Such an article would be unthinkable today – and so much the better. Deconstruction has begun, and women – and even some men – are calling out the inequalities, dissatisfaction and suffering that make up the banal reality of straight sex. But there remains strong resistance, because sexism is so embedded.

   In addition, we have to discuss an extremely perverse mechanism that pushes us to blame women: if they don't feel pleasure, it must be their fault. They obviously aren't relaxed enough, they're blocked in some way, or have unresolved issues. They are also obviously too 'clitoris-dependent'.

O de G   'Too clitoris-dependent': that's absurd! The clitoris is the pleasure organ par excellence. More than 10,000 nerve endings. And it should be ignored? For too long, female sexuality has been misrepresented by theorists such as those in the medical profession. Personally, I've suffered because of these ideas. I read *Feminine Sexuality* when I was on the point of discovering my sexuality. I was convinced, as Françoise Dolto said – and Sigmund Freud before her – that, in order to become a 'real' woman, I would have to, one day, stop rubbing and stroking myself, and learn to feel pleasure from penetration – although it hurt me! Deconstructing these ideas took me time.

SE   The history of the clitoris is also very revealing about the power society exerts on our pleasure. Discovered in the sixteenth century, and recognised for its erogenous properties, the clitoris was *removed* from anatomy books by natalist politicians. They went as far as considering it to be dangerous.

O de G   More masturbation, less procreation...

SE   That's right. It was only in 1998 that, thanks to work by Australian urologist Helen O'Connell, a representation of the clitoris worthy of the name was put forward. While for the penis, representations have never been lacking!

MP   Sex is political. But the way it is represented is still archaic. Men play the leading role: they are powerful and desirable, they decide what goes and enforce it. That's what society teaches us. From that moment onwards, women are trapped: their oppressors are desirable, and they define what good behaviour must look like. Thereafter, heterosexual love for women can only go wrong, since they are exploited, not fully listened to. They are guilt-tripped and often unhappy.

SE   This pattern seems so entrenched. How can we transform it?

MP   Deconstructing and asking questions about our desires allows us to call out the underlying toxic mechanisms. Individual reflection is important, but I'm convinced that change will be brought about through joint action, books, fiction and voluntary organisations. Women are the ones grappling with these questions, because they are the victims. Men ought to support them and be their allies.

O de G   Everyone would benefit.

MP   Who isn't in favour of a fairer world? Men must learn that penetration is one possible choice, but it's not the be-all and end-all of heterosexual sex. It's not mandatory. It's up to them to talk to their partners, to listen to them, to learn what they enjoy and what they desire. They must no longer assume that only their desires count; they must stop imposing those desires. It's a question of social justice and democracy at the end of the day: men and women deserve the same rights and the same joy. We must fight together to ensure equality throughout our love lives and sex lives, and to reach a place where happiness and pleasure are equally shared at last.

SE   What works would you highlight on the subject of sexuality?

MP   I would suggest reading Mireille Havet, a poet from the early twentieth century who moved in Parisian lesbian circles during the interwar years and wrote a beautiful diary. She was friends with Apollinaire, Cocteau and Colette, and she writes about her lavish life and her homosexual lovers in a very beautiful and open way.

I would also recommend Mélanie Fazi's essential book on asexuality, *Nous qui n'existons pas*.

Another one to read is *Sortir de l'hétérosexualité*, by Juliet Drouar. The author and trans activist reflects on the possibility of questioning the oppressiveness of standard thinking.

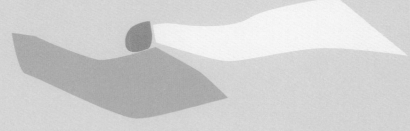

Chapter 6

Online shopping
for partners

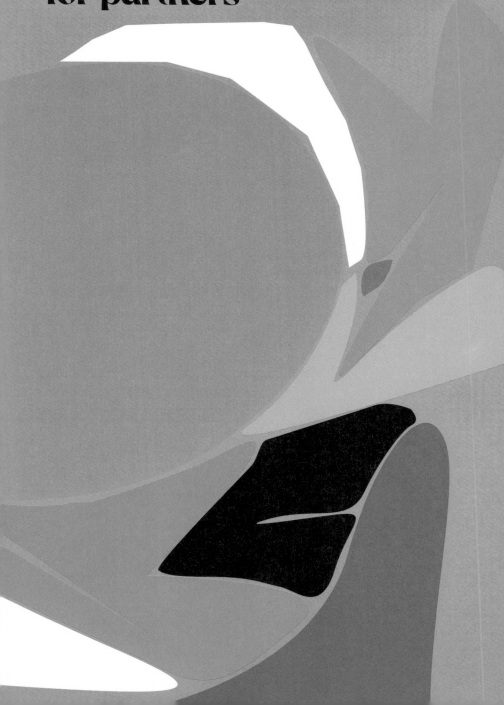

Monday 20 September 2021

9.30am

I open one eye and remove my sleep mask. The sun streams on to my bed. Through the window, I can see blue and green, brown and flashy orange; I can hear magpies squabbling, woodpigeons cooing. The weekend was spent working. I stretch and feel a twitching sensation in my back and thigh muscles. The autumn is rushing by; I feel I'm not making the most of it. I want to be in early summer at the seaside, snogging someone, pressing my wet swimsuit against a man's torso, taking a late-afternoon siesta in the long grass, resting my head on someone's shoulder. I want to share my sensuality, to have sex with someone and discover a new body. That would be 'making the most of it'!

Beach-wise, it's doable. I live in a village not far from the sea in Brittany. Meeting a man to lie close to as the tide rises around our entwined bodies, on the other hand, is more complicated. People living round here are mostly elderly and families... Hunky, unattached thirty-five-year olds tend not to hang out in the countryside. Perhaps I can do some searching on dating apps?

As a little girl, I was very short-sighted. I opted for laser-eye surgery aged twenty-five, but in my teens, I simply couldn't survive without my glasses. I used to imagine how ghastly my life would have been if I'd lived in prehistoric times – or, at least, before corrective glasses had been invented. Likewise, this morning, lying in bed, I shiver at all the social niceties I would have had to endure to meet someone willing to dive with me into the sea off the coast of Brittany, and then into my bed, if Tinder, Happn, OkCupid, Bumble *et al.* hadn't been invented.

Despite the current pervasive sense of perma-crisis around all things environmental, social and health-based, the feeling of the sun slowly working its way up my thigh reminds me how lucky I am to live in the age of the booty call. I am free to express my desire for sex – and, by spending a bit of time scanning profiles, I'll probably be able to satisfy my needs.

I feel all the more fortunate to be a woman. In prehistoric times, my short-sightedness would have been my undoing; I may have ended up in the jaws of a sabre-toothed tiger. Even in more recent times, I would probably have been burned at the stake, stoned to death or had my clitoris doused in carbolic acid by one of Dr Kellogg's disciples – or worse – simply for being a woman with desires.

11.30am

Still in bed, and now the sun is kissing my belly. I've just reactivated and updated my Tinder profile. The photos were only three years old but, bizarrely, now I'm over thirty-five, three years seems a lifetime. I feel obliged to be honest online about the current state of my skin, my crow's feet and grey hairs.

It took me two attempts.

Initially, I didn't overthink it, and put together a true-to-form profile. The first photo showed me with my cat, illuminated by a sunbeam. Above us hung a David Shrigley painting with the words 'Life is very good' and a blue galloping horse. The other photos showed me horse-riding or in a swimsuit on an island off the Brittany coast. There were also some 'official' portraits of me attending conferences or other events. I tried to portray the different facets of my life. My biography read: 'Freedom, love, sorority. And also: desire, intensity, enthusiasm.'

Then I had second thoughts about the pictures. I tried something else, a really punchy presentation of myself, with beautiful photos taken on film sets when I was performing. Me, riding a motorbike, my nipples erect beneath a white cotton T-shirt... me, stretched out on a Le Corbusier chair, clad only in a white leather harness... The photos are small and surrounded by a broad black mount, so you can only just make them out. They are at least five years old, so I mix them up with more recent photos of my face, in a spirit of honesty, as though someone might accuse me of mis-selling goods, as though I need to justify the state of my skin.

1pm

I really ought to get up. But the algorithms of these apps are well designed. First up are the most attractive guys – the good-job, good-looking, 'high-end' types. Argh.

'High-end types'...

I soon get the hang of the apps. The men I scroll through are no longer people, they're profiles, and I judge them on spelling, originality and good taste, with a practised and pitiless eye. I gauge their sexual capital, to quote the sociologist who studies relationships, Eva Illouz. The apps reveal the way I discriminate in sexual and emotional dealings. I realise that when I want to share a sexual adventure, I hunt out someone from my social class.

Ooh, a 'super like'. Nice-looking boy. Footballer. I turn him down. I've already experienced a one-night stand with a footballer. In bed, the guy played hands-free.

As I continue to swipe, I am struck by something. Over half the men opting to write something underneath their photos state they are looking for 'no-drama'. What an unrealistic expectation! Is it the virtual nature of apps that makes these men lose sight of the reality of intimate relationships? This 'no-drama' approach suggests the hope that a woman will agree with them: that they will understand each other, without needing any recourse to words, without discussing things, or negotiating them; that it's all self-evident. Who doesn't like fluid relationships, ease of communication? Me too! I dream of simplicity! But I also know it comes at a price. One of opening up to the other person, of listening to each other, of showing emotional courage, and allowing yourself to be vulnerable. Much as I've always harboured soppy hopes (of meeting a physio who's starred in *Top Chef*, for example) I feel it's pretty naive for men in their thirties or forties to be looking for a sexual and emotional relationship that's hassle-free and perfect. Who really experiences that? What family relationship, professional partnership or long-term friendship doesn't, at some time, go through moments of tension and disagreement, where you have to negotiate a lot of hassle to realign and regain your former harmony? Is a life of love really not worth the effort in the eyes of all these men?

As I land upon the umpteenth 'no-drama' profile, I wonder if this condition isn't indicative of laziness to some extent... Yes, these men are setting limits; they don't want arguments, they probably believe that life is too short to spend it squabbling. However, when you're a straight man, refusing to make the effort to resolve the slightest disagreement with your partner smacks of sitting tight, arms crossed, and leaving it up to women to nurture the relationship from A to Z. Because if they're going to please this man and his no-drama wishes, women are going to have to use their emotional antennae at every turn, and endeavour at all times (often while in a state of anxiety) to understand him. They will have to make their own adjustments in order to decipher the implicit situation and grasp what hasn't been spoken out loud. If they want to express their needs, make requests, they will need to take endless precautions for fear of upsetting him. In short, they will have to throw a lot of energy – and tact – into nurturing the relationship – and, ultimately, the man. To the detriment of their own emotional and personal needs. A friend of mine said she calls men who have a phobia of being involved in any hassle 'emotional slackers'. I love this expression![30]

2pm

QED: Ironically, this question of wanting things to be 'no-drama' has irritated me. On the plus side, it means I've got out of bed. Under the shower, using Coué's conscious auto-suggestion method, I remember the positive aspect of apps, the reason I've signed up to them again: the lovers! My favourites were those I met while travelling abroad. Not so much for the encounter – often short-lived, celebratory and too alcohol-fuelled – but for the aftermath. I would return home, thousands of kilometres away, carrying the excitement of a new beginning. I kept up this sexual energy through my images and words, sent by WhatsApp. These men were in London, Berlin, Moscow, and I wrote to them about my body and my desire for sex in texts, poems – even songs! I turned these feelings into drawings. I photographed them; I would go and fondle the buttocks of statues and reveal my own in churchyards.

And then I got hold of some accessories: a waterproof case for my smartphone, a selfie-stick, a wide-angle lens so I could take full-length shots, a macro lens to film my skin, rainbow-coloured bulbs. I filmed, edited, added music, and was passionately engrossed for hours on end. The lovers gradually disappeared as I threw myself into my creations. After several months of this creative process, I was so proud of my productions that I wanted to make more. And not just for those few men who came into my life like ships in the night...

That's why I decided to make an alternative porn film.

Wednesday 6 October 2021

4pm

I've been naive in thinking that hot images of me set against a black background would keep weirdos at bay. There are desperate people out there: first, they do Google Image searches using my photos to find out my name; second, they trawl through my social media accounts; third, they send me suspicious messages. There's even one guy who sent me a photo of his tackle, barely covered by my first book![31] I'm delighted to know he's used these pages (co-authored with Stéphanie) as a penis sheath.

Bar that surprise, I've been contacted by endless male 'candidates' who want 'to be porn stars'. I replied politely to the first few, giving them my standard advice: start by creating content yourself, make it available on OnlyFans, and gently let yourself into the business. I stopped replying when one of them brutally responded: 'You frustrated bitch, go fuck yourself with your punk pussy hair.' That ended up in my local police station, where I filed a formal complaint for sexist slander. All in all, anything *but* stimulating exchanges...

Although it might seem a surprising comparison, I see similarities between my premenstrual syndrome and the reactions I get on the internet as a woman affirming herself as a sex subject. Every month for the last twenty-five years, I am moody, messed up; the monkey in my head tries to persuade me I'm too this and not enough that, that I need to change all my life... And suddenly, surprise surprise, I get my period! The same is true every time I appear on the internet as a woman living her sexuality freely. Whether I'm talking publicly about my work as a film director, or looking for an intimate partner, I'm expecting dialogue, opportunities, encounters... and surprise, surprise, a black trail of insults follows behind!

9pm

While working, I came across a video in my archives of a porn star I admire. I was so impressed by her, I had taken some screen captures. She was dealing with the problem that all X-rated actors have in controlling what happens to their images:

'I'm tired of seeing my image used everywhere without my permission. When you work in the porn industry, you generally sign a very unfavourable contract in which you authorise the production team not only to sell your image under their name, but also to sell it on to third parties without letting you know, without your consent and without paying you any extra. [...] They can put me on the cover of a Polish magazine without [me] having any inkling of what's going on.'[32]

This video struck a chord because it put into words a discomfort I felt one year after my first film as a performer came out. This short-length movie[33] was directed by Lucie Blush in my home, in my intimate space, one Sunday morning. I made love to a man on my bed and then in my sitting room. When I agreed to filming, Lucie Blush's work was solely available on her subscription-only website. Being protected behind a paywall was a *sine qua non* for me to take part. To pay for porn made by a woman was, in itself, a militant gesture; I believed I was stripping off only in front of people as convinced as I am that you can be a woman and enjoy your body freely. However, one year on, the film was available in full on an X-rated platform, free of charge. All you needed to do was click on the 'I'm over eighteen years old' button to watch it. What's more, it was referenced with the hashtags: #smalltits, #teen, #redhead...

I reported the pirated video to the platform. Waste of effort. Once a porn film is out there, removing it from circulation is almost impossible. Even when the producer decides to take a scene offline at the request of a performer, the film has normally already been reposted a dozen or more times. As revolting as it is, it is wishful thinking to try to control your image in the world of porn.

Is this issue limited to the X-rated world? I don't think so. The very fact that I have screen captures among my files of an X-rated performer expressing her views on the profession is a problem in itself. Perhaps one day she will want to remove this opinion from her YouTube channel. Nonetheless, I'll still have my trace of it. Or, perhaps, YouTube will one day decide to censor comments made on sex and pornography. It's not such a dystopian concept when you see what a problem social networks have with sexuality. On Instagram, we are obliged to censor our nipples and even write 'segsuality' instead of 'sexuality' to avoid being shadow-banned! If the platform were to remove such videos, the fact that I've kept an archive could be interesting, advantageous.

Beyond all these moral judgements, there are some constant truths. We live in an era of exponential reproductivity of images on the internet. And sexual images depicting young women are the ones most at risk of going viral. As a woman, living your life online implies that your content can be dug up, or even brought back to light from long-forgotten corners. It can then be re-used, decontextualized, pirated and used against you, and could give rise to waves of trolling. Our online texts and images can also allow us to meet people, to bring awareness to tens of thousands of individuals about a particular cause, to make others laugh, to find love...That's (online) life!

Thursday 4 November 2021

3pm

I'm on my terrace, wrapped in a blanket. Having put my book aside for a brief moment, I discover I've been matched with a man I like the look of. His name is Rayan, he's twenty-eight years old, and he's a junior doctor in neurology. He's left me a message, barely ten words in all, but amusing – and, what's more, there are no spelling mistakes. A smile on my lips, I suggest we meet for coffee soon. He's in Brest, which is more than a stone's throw away, but doable. The guy tells me: 'I'd like to have more than just a coffee with you.' That sets my heart racing.

I reply that if he wants to sext, I'm free all afternoon. Rayan calls me there and then! I don't pick up; I'm somewhat timid about phones. He tries again. Alright. I pick up the call. I hear his deep voice telling me I'm giving him a serious hard-on. I'm not too sure what else we talk about, to be honest, but we speak for a long, long time. He makes me laugh, and his voice excites me. His French is strongly accented, and he tells me he only arrived in France three months ago. When we hang up, I'm super turned on. Via WhatsApp, he sends me photos of his cock, and I'm delighted. I try to take a couple of photos of my breasts, my hand between my thighs. I realise I'm a bit rusty; the pictures aren't up to much.

The sexual tension mounts. I'm boiling over; my mind wanders to a junior doctor's bedroom, at the West of the West of Europe. That evening, he calls back, this time on video. He's naked, stretched out on the bed, holding his cock. He spits into his palm and jerks off vigorously; he calls me baby. Ha ha! I love it! He wants to see my pussy. When I show him, he says: 'Now that's a pussy!'

I'm totally hooked.

Monday 8 November 2021

3pm

For four days, we haven't let up, Rayan and I. We send each other photos, voice messages. I've climaxed more times than I can remember. I start touching myself as soon as I get back home; he fires me up so much. Between the burning waves of libido and urgent orgasms, I wonder whether this is what's missing in my life. A 100 per cent virtual relationship. There is something simultaneously free and reassuring about the situation.

Somebody desires me, intensely; I feel myself living to the full. Yet this person is not going to interfere in my life, bring on massive jealous fits, or leave pee around my toilet bowl. I have the pleasure of sexuality without the discomfort that otherness can trigger.

11.30pm

I find myself day-dreaming about 'making my life' with Rayan. Thanks to the intense desire, my female brain, nurtured on fairy tales, has begun to fantasise about a possible love story. I'm seeing Stéphanie tomorrow. I'll talk to her about it. I feel I have a topic for feminist reflection.

Tuesday 30 November 2021

11am

It turns out that Stéphanie is busy for the next few days. We're going to chat over video. 'Being there' (her words) for her two teenage daughters is still her priority, and it seems one of them is currently in need of lots of TLC. I understand and respect her decision 100 per cent.

I've started telling Stéphanie about 'the subject of Rayan' by text. She says she's really pleased for me, but I sense a level of mistrust on her part, as though she's saying, 'Let's see where it all goes before weighing in.'

4pm

Stéphanie and I have opposite ideas about digital meet-ups. Is it a generational thing? Stéphanie has told me about her own usage of dating sites – and she's suspended them since. She has always been exceptionally cautious: no exchange of erotic or pornographic pictures by either party, something of a veiled approach:

'At the time, working as a journalist for a daily newspaper, I was, to some extent, obliged to be careful about my image. But even without this professional background, I've always been concerned about the traces

I may or may not be leaving behind me. The way you build your profile – photos of yourself wearing a harness, etc. – are out of the question for me, because I need to be able to keep a barrier between my intimacy and extimacy – by that, I mean the intimate part of myself I choose to make public. I would feel completely insecure by being categorised as a sexual subject. Even if I am.'

For my part, I feel that my intimate sphere is not embodied in what I show others, even if it's very easy to see me naked on the internet. Photos of me wearing a harness, bare-breasted, are a powerful affirmation: I can love my body separately from being observed by men; I want to have a free and creative sexuality. A similar approach to slut walks:[34] the shame I am told I should be feeling, I convert into pride!

Indeed, showing myself intimately is a political move for me. The more that people try to dissuade us by insulting us and humiliating us, the more it pushes me to defy ambient sexism. To demonstrate that I will only do what suits me.

And to take what I'm feeling to its furthest extreme, my real intimacy is anywhere but in my nudity or in the sex I show on the internet. It's in my vulnerability, my weak moments, my sometimes complicated relationship with my body; it resides in my fear of screwing up when making love, in my anxiety when I no longer want to have sex. Basically, it's in all these details that say more about me and my background than the shape of my nipples or how I shave my pubic hair!

6.10pm

Throwing myself into a long relationship with Rayan... Seen from the standpoint of a woman in full control of her life and her desires, it would not make sense. And yet, these sorts of thoughts return to me once in a while. A need to see myself in an 'ideal relationship' alongside an 'ideal man' – without knowing, really, what that adjective means.

As far back as I can remember, I have nurtured my fantasies. I have launched myself into all sorts of love stories with immense pleasure. From nursery school, throughout my education and beyond, I have loved.

To think of a man is – still today – a sweet joy. It is through validation from a man that a young girl is supposed to find her value. In children's storybooks, fairy tales, this is what she is told: men become masters of the world; women fulfill themselves through romance. As a young girl, this need for male validation set my heart racing. I *had* to be loved. Share my daily world with a boy. Still today, despite years of deconstructing and realisations, I love dreaming about being with a man, just like you suck on a sweet.

According to Stéphanie, most of us, heterosexual women, start off life weighed down by our need to fulfill ourselves via our couple – our need to make a man happy. It's what we're taught, what society hands on to us as a model via a wide variety of channels (advertisements, cinema, TV, literature, etc.).

And yes, over the past few years, things have started to change. More and more often, I read accounts on social media written by single women who are happy in their own skins. Lesbian couples' visibility is also gradually building up a counterpoint.

We won't be able to change everything with a snap of our fingers, Stéphanie has just reminded me; we won't be able to change *ourselves* with a snap of our fingers. But do let's continue deconstructing. By reflecting, first of all, on what is best for us, we're on the right track.

9.30pm

I absolutely can dream about making my life with Rayan, given that I know where I stand in my relationship. For the moment, I am aware that this dream is a fairy tale and I accept it as thus. In my real life, I acknowledge that Rayan is a prop for my libido. It suits me like that.

Deconstructing my daydreams – I realise today – is essential with online dating. The scenarios I grew up with were focused on love as salvation, a coming-together that guarantees perfect and unchangeable happiness. Losing myself in these dreams with a sense of destiny each time I have a new hook-up is not a fair use of my mental time and creative energy. I have to stop investing myself emotionally in so many of my crushes!

10pm

Agreed to meet Rayan tomorrow, to have a drink and see what happens. If I were listening to my inner self, I'd skip this step, but it does offer a sort of guarantee. You can get to know each other's voices, smells, gestures, through the chemistry of each other's bodies and words. Stéphanie told me she'd had one or two disappointing experiences when it came to meeting up in real life. It simply didn't work out. As though the other person, all of a sudden, no longer evoked any feelings in her.

For my part, that's never happened. I consider this stage more a way of enhancing my desire still further before jumping in feet first.

Wednesday 1 December 2021

1.30am

I can't sleep. Rayan wasn't free this evening, but he's sent me some sexts that set me burning with desire. I am mesmerised! It's hard to calm myself down.

And what if, at last, things between us really hit the jackpot? After all, that option exists.

3.30am

I've reread my most recent exchanges with Stéphanie. I think it's brought me back down to earth. Perhaps the flare of my libido means I tend to overreact. So, I have everything to gain by going to this meet-up, unencumbered by my expectations! I ought to concentrate on how good it will feel to discover his body and for him to discover mine... How we will laugh, tell each other our life stories, rather than asking myself if we're going to get on, if we'll want to spend more and more time together, etc. OK, I'm going to try to sleep on it all.

6.30pm

A couple of almost shy exchanges with Rayan since this morning. Perhaps he's less keen; perhaps, at the end of the day, he's rather reserved. Maybe he doesn't enjoy real-life meetings. I prefer it when he desires me blindly, when he tells me so. When he excites me. All the same, so much the better. I am calmer. And able to tell myself that there is no question of sleeping with him if I don't feel 100 per cent in the mood. A somewhat sad thought, thinking back to all my hook-ups when I was younger, when I found myself snogging a guy, or even going further, because he wasn't bad, because we were both turned on... even if, at the end of the day, I didn't really fancy him. Aged thirty-nine, I'm going to promise myself those days are over. I am listening to myself.

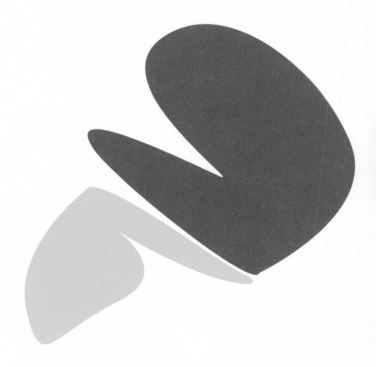

The art of safe hook-ups

Online dating apps occupy an important place in our emotional and sexual lives. In the United States, they are the most common way people pair up, accounting for 40 per cent of online coupling![35] It can be more risky surfing in these zones – as for everything else – if you are a women; all the more so if you also belong to an ethnic or sexual minority. So, here is some advice to take advantage of the potential offered by these apps in as safe a way as possible.

CHOOSE YOUR PHOTOS WITH CARE

When you set up a profile on a dating app, use photos of yourself that you don't use anywhere else online. If you use the same photo on Instagram and Tinder, a simple reverse-image search on Google Images will allow anyone to find you on social media based on your Tinder profile pictures.

STICK TO COMMUNICATING WITHIN THE DATING APP

When chatting with your matches, stick to the in-house messaging service of the dating app until you're sure you want to keep talking to this person. OK, it's a bit less practical, but it's safer.

IF IN DOUBT, BLOCK THEM!

Trust your instincts: if you're not getting the vibe from someone, or from a situation, say goodbye. And if the match is behaving inappropriately towards you, don't think twice: block them – and report them.

'HI; I'M GOING OUT'

Tell those closest to you where and when you're meeting your date for the first time. Make sure you meet somewhere safe and public, such as a park, café or bar. And, importantly: make sure you have an independent means of transport from your match.

CONSIDER STARTING WITH A VIDEO CALL

If you're into impromptu sex and want to jump straight in with both feet on your date, you can suggest having a video call just before you set off. Hearing the other person's voice and seeing how they react on screen can enable you to confirm whether you feel a good vibe or not.

DON'T CONNECT WITH SUSPECT PROFILES

There are con artists on dating apps, as there are everywhere. Sadly, some of them are even renowned, like the so-called 'Tinder Swindler', whose misdeeds were the subject of a true crime documentary on Netflix. Here are some examples of suspect behaviour that might alert you:

- They don't have a bio and have only published one photo.
- They are pressuring you to give them your number or to speak to them outside the app before you're ready to.
- They ask for your address on the pretext of sending you a present.
- They suddenly disappear from the site, then reappear under a different name.

- They consistently give vague replies to specific questions.
- They come across as exaggeratedly romantic far too early.
- They ask for financial help for a personal and urgent reason.

NEVER SEND MONEY

Avoid any financial transactions with someone you hardly know. Don't lend them money, don't send them gift cards, don't give out any information about your accounts, and don't trust any investment advice.

DON'T REVEAL TOO MUCH ABOUT YOURSELF

Keep your place of work and your address secret until you feel you can trust them. It's also recommended to keep your surname secret until after your first meeting.

To sext or not to sext? That is the question!

Everybody sexts... or almost everyone![36] When consensual, sexting is a joyful practice that's good for the ego, libido and sexual communication. All the same, it's important to be aware that as far as sexting is concerned, there is no such thing as zero risk.

HACKING YOUR WAY THROUGH THE JUNGLE OF ONLINE DATING

Did you know that nearly 25 per cent of people who receive sexts share them with others?[37] This isn't just down to insensitivity or carelessness. Some people do this out of pure spite: revenge porn, for example, or hacking – as happened to a number of high profile women in

2014 when nude pictures of them were revealed following a security failure in the cloud. Things like this can have profound consequences on the lives and mental health of their victims. The fight against cybercrime is ongoing, but it is still difficult to be 100 per cent sure about the confidentiality of our steamy messages.

BEYOND RAPE CULTURE

When the topic of sexting comes up for a women, we are advised, more often than not. to avoid participating in any such intimate exchanges. It's customary, in fact, in our patriarchal societies to urge women to protect themselves against potential crimes against them. It seems to be preferable to prevent us from doing what we enjoy rather than making public space – whether real or virtual – more secure, and educating and punishing our aggressors. When a women is unfortunate enough to be the victim of a cybercrime, they find themselves not only faced with the initial act of violence, but also the insinuation that, by sexting, they 'brought it upon themselves'.

Let's remember and underline the fact that cyber criminals, whether they are hackers, spreaders of revenge porn, or unscrupulous partners, are the *only* ones to blame here. We are never guilty for having wanted to be part of an exchange or interaction, or for enjoying our own bodies.

IT'S UP TO YOU TO PLAY… OR NOT!

The decision whether or not to sext falls to you alone. It depends on your own personal relationship with your nudity (is nudity a very intimate thing for you? Are you reserved or more relaxed where your body is concerned?), and also how you feel about the risks involved.

If you wish to engage in the pleasure of sexting, here is some advice for doing so in the safest way possible:

Choose your playing field

Rather than exchanging NSFW messages on Instagram, WhatsApp or Snapchat, choose an app that you *don't* use to communicate with your nearest and dearest – or with work! Best of all, download an app to use exclusively for sexting and nothing else. If you've got an iPhone, try Privates, an app that allows you to programme an expiry date for photos and prevent screen shots. On Android, there is Signal, which also allows you to deactivate screenshots. Signal has the added advantage of end-to-end encryption, which offers you greater protection against computer hackers.

Frame your photos with care

When you take an intimate photo, avoid including your face in the frame, or ensure that only a minimum part of it can be seen: for example, your mouth. You can also play around with wearing a mask, hiding your eyes behind your hands, covering your face with your hair, using backlighting... There are endless creative options to choose from.

> ▶ NB: if you are tattooed, as well as hiding your face, don't photograph any of your tattoos that are visible when you're dressed. You can cover them up with a scarf, your hair, etc.

And now... bring on the fun!

If you have decided you would like to engage in sexting, here are some ideas to explore.

DO YOU TALK DIRTY?

A very effective and low-risk way of sexting is to count on the power of words. A well-balanced text can fill your sexting partner with passion in less time than it takes to snap a suitable selfie... But we have to admit, dirty talk can be intimidating. The fault lies in the prudishness surrounding sex that expects us only to groan inarticulately during intercourse. We don't have the habit of juggling words of pleasure, or communicating in a daring and playful manner while lovemaking. If the thought of improvising dirty talk in your chats scares you, we have an alternative plan. It's a bit like the idea of thesis, antithesis and synthesis, but adapted for sexting:

1. You state what you would like to do: 'I really want to XXX your XXX.'

2. You ask permission: 'May I XXX your XXX?' Then you wait for a 'yes'.

3. Once they have said 'yes', you describe the action in more detail: 'I will XXXX your XXX from XXX to XXX, XXXly.' Then you check: 'Do you like how I XXX your XXX?'

4. Round off: 'Mmmm, I love XXXing your XXX.'

GRAB THEM BY THE ... EAR

A tad more engaging than sticking to the written word, yet with fewer implications than photos: voice messages. They are both mysterious when you've never met in the flesh and extremely intimate; it's a real surprise to hear an unknown person's voice whispering their desires in your ear. You could record the sounds of your pleasure while you're touching yourself, or you could verbally let them know what you would like them to do to you...

NOW FOR YOUR NUDES

We all remember the first unsolicited nude photo we received: in the main, we were (very) young, and it was a stranger's dick pic, sent on a social network that was supposed to be family-friendly. We felt disgusted, we were shocked... it was a violation. Whatever our identity or gender, the last thing anyone wants today is to impose their sexuality on others. So it's very important to ask your partner whether they would like to receive nude photos from you, and to check regularly that they still want to receive them, especially in the daytime during working hours. Once you have agreed this, you can enjoy the art of creating nudes.

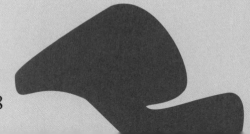

Ramp things up a notch

Sending nude photos is a bit like choreographing a striptease show. Start with suggestive images that only just allow your body to be distinguished. If the light is good, don't hesitate to make use of close-up shots: mouth, tongue, wet fingers, erect nipples under a piece of material... Wait until they ask for more, or even beg you! Then raise the temperature by being even more explicit.

Stay in the moment

Resist the temptation to prepare a whole series of pre-sequenced nudes, and try to resist retouching your images. What makes it hot is being spontaneous, and genuinely and immediately sharing! By improvising your nudes based on your partner's reactions, you are letting them know that you're living the actual moment, in real time, taking pleasure in the process with them.

CONCENTRATE ON YOUR TASTES AND DESIRES

Not only does sexting offer the excitement of sharing something with a partner, it also brings you the safe intimacy of solo sex. Before moving on to an IRL meeting, sexting can provide an excellent means of communicating what you enjoy. When you take a nude photo of yourself, take advantage of the chance to explain how you would like someone to move their hand over your body, your genitals. Share what positions appeal to you... say which words and gestures turn you on. This will raise the temperature even before there is a skin-on-skin meeting.

30 Extract from a text initially published on Olympe's blog and edited for this book.
31 Estournet, S. & de Gê, O. 2021, *Jouir est un sport de combat*, Larousse, Paris.
32 This performer has stopped working in the porn business and, in order to ease her transition, doesn't want to have her name published.
33 Blush, L. 2016, *Un beau dimanche*, Self production.
34 Slut walks are marches against sexual assaults and violence, and any stigmatisation of victims whose look is deemed 'provocative'. The first slut walk took place in 2011 in Toronto, Canada.
35 According to a Stanford study published in 2019, around 40 per cent of American couples now first meet online.
36 Out of 870 people who took part in a study by Drexel University in 2015, 88 per cent said they had already sexted: 'Most adults are sexting and that may not be a bad thing,' Drexel News, 10 August 2015 (https://drexel.edu/news/archive/2015/august/sexting-study).
37 This is according to a 2016 study involving nearly 6,000 single adult respondents: Garcia, J. R., *et al.* July 2016, 'Sexting among singles in the USA: prevalence of sending, receiving and sharing sexual messages and images,' *Sexual Health*.

Chapter 7

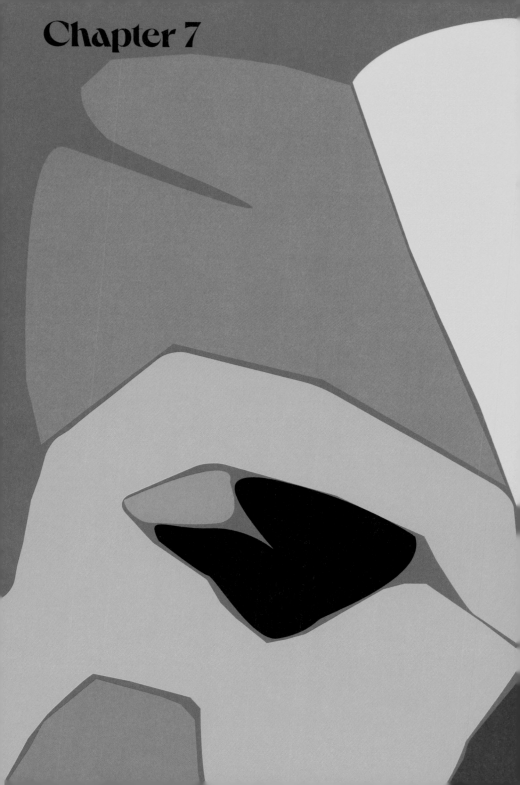

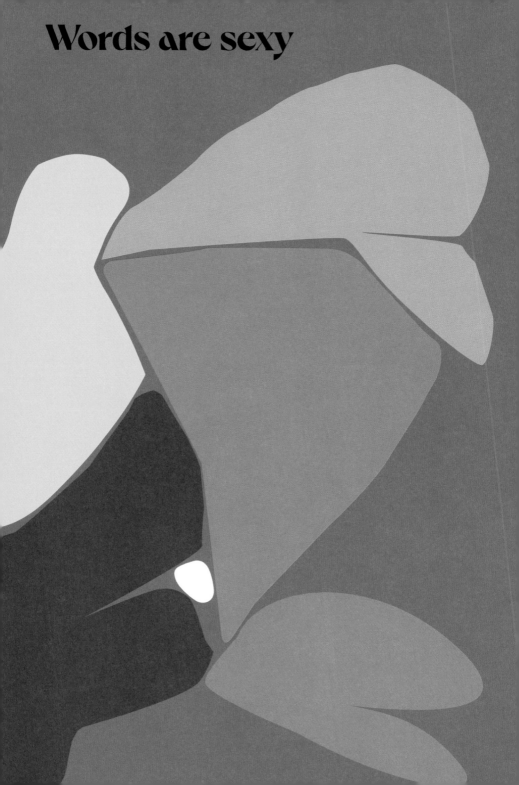

Words are sexy

It was the words that stayed with me ...

Like Olympe, who grew-up in a home with no TV, I discovered sexuality from books. Not really through proper literature though, but via photo-novels. Back in the 1980s, people still read photo-novels and they were – really – pornographic: the pages of text alternated with full-page photographs featuring wide-shot scenes as well as close-ups of genitals and seemingly hedonistic young women.

In 'photo-novel' you've got the word 'novel': characters (caricatures, in the case in point), intrigue, separate chapters, progression and resolution. The words work in conjunction with the images to create an unreal atmosphere. You look, read and look again... I was hypnotised by the double erotic effect of the mere existence of this pornographic object.

What was I left with when I closed the book? More than the images, it was the words that stayed with me: the dirty talk, the word-based erotic relationship, the situational descriptions. In short, the storyline.

Photo-novels have since disappeared, and pornographic films with a storyline constitute a fringe category on free X-rated platforms – as though plot-based porn was in itself kinky. 'Traditional' writing for the porn film industry before the 1990s included a psychological or at least a creative approach. This has more or less disappeared in hardcore porn. The storytelling consists now in some pseudo-realistic plot lines, simplified into tropes: 'baby-sitter', 'family', or 'college'. Less creativity, more efficiency.

That the text of these pornographic photo-novels seemed more transgressive to me than the photographs (which were, nevertheless, super-explicit), perhaps comes down to the fact that – personally – the act of saying something amounts to intimate participation. By uttering the words, the characters are not merely pawns and part of a process. They are affirming themselves as full-blown sexual beings, and fully aware of it. They claim this status. And that is really transgressive.

Identify and share

But life isn't a photo-novel, and it can be difficult to express oneself in the context of shared sexuality; to simply say what you're feeling. Today, we're still expected to keep quiet about our bodies, especially anything to do with our genitals and pleasure. In porn films, men invariably remain silent until the crucial moment (when they eventually grunt something along the lines of, 'Come here, you little slut,' or 'You like that, don't you, dirty whore.'). The women's voices, meanwhile, become ever more shrill to signify their desire and, thereby, their lover's talent in bringing them to orgasm. It's hard to see oneself depicted in these gendered stereotypes.

For my part I realised how conventional my ways of expressing myself during sexual intercourse were in a shared moment with a man who kept on moaning. The thought *Just like a girl* went coursing through my mind. *My lover is behaving like a girl.* I couldn't get the idea out of my head between dates with him. Was this man really what he declared – heterosexual? Was he about to spring something on me that 'straight people don't do' – such as asking me to penetrate him, for example? That's what I was turning over in my mind, simply because this man didn't follow the stereotype of buttoned-up silence during our lovemaking, as expected of his sex.

To be capable of expressing our sexual and pleasure-related desires – and equally to be able to express that something hurts, that we are uncomfortable – seems to me, today, to be a prerequisite if we are to live our sexuality to the full. We must identify our desires, share what makes us uneasy. Find the right words. Feel free to say them. I try to do this. I don't always succeed. Sometimes, I just don't *know* what I'm feeling, what I want, what I don't want. Sometimes, I fear offending my partner, by starting to talk too soon, coming across as selfish. But there is one thing I know after all these years: if I don't try to put my feelings into words, my partner cannot guess what they are. By trying to explain it, I'm giving us a chance to succeed.

Starting point: consent (yippee!)

The starting point for any relationship: consent. Fiction, especially cinema, has constructed a powerful stereotype: the love affair that appears to involve instant physical recognition of the other person, with no need for any verbal exchanges. This stereotype suggests we understand each other thanks to our hormones and the magic of love – or the effect of the full moon, or the alignment of the planets – and that we will, therefore, make all the correct moves, in a sort of perfectly rhythmic and harmonious dance. Smouldering glances, passionate kisses... (At this point, the camera pans away from the two blissful figures, ending the shot on a window looking out on a peaceful night.) There is no need for words, this stereotype tells us, as if words are blunt instruments and using them implies you might be unsure about the other person's desire.

Cinema adheres to its own storytelling requirements, and those don't have to be realistic. Just as you're not going to cling on for dear life to a runaway bus because your lover is inside and you know the brakes have failed, a love story as depicted in films (I'm talking here about pornographic and non-pornographic films!) shouldn't dictate our behaviour. Desire isn't a given, and from that first kiss through to a slap on the backside, via stroking or undressing the other person, it's not open season. It's much better to make a suggestion, and be sure of your partner's wishes. You believing they are willing is not the same as them being willing. If there is any shadow of a doubt, if any movement hints at discomfort, don't wait to ask: 'Is it OK if I touch you there?'; 'Can I take your top off?' If the other person responds evasively or timidly, or says nothing at all, it's best to calmly press the pause button. You can talk about something else, or do something else – remember that there shouldn't be any expectation of what will happen. Just because we are turned on, doesn't mean our partners owe us anything. Olympe and I often joke about it: the bathroom isn't out of bounds! If I'm turned on and my partner isn't on the same wavelength, I'm free to find a quiet place, bring my heightened excitement down a notch or two, masturbate if I feel like it. I certainly shouldn't put any pressure on my partner.

Of course, there's a basic principle of reciprocity: my partner certainly shouldn't put any pressure on me. And when we are playing, say, a domination game, we will have discussed it together beforehand to explain our desires, and either of us should be able to say at any moment, during the fun, *No, not that, not there, not now*, as well as *Yes, I love that*.

By anticipating the action, by providing subtitles, our words create an additional link between us that anchors us. And – in addition – isn't that what we are all looking for: feeling in touch with one another and reassured?

Towards our limits, and beyond!

But in order to be attentive towards the other person and able to express myself, I have first and foremost to be attentive towards myself. I need to be capable of knowing what I want and what I don't want, of naming my limits (which change from one moment to the next; there was a certain thing I didn't want to do half an hour ago, and now I'm gagging for it!).

I've said it already: it's not easy.

This awareness of what is and isn't good for me at a particular moment should be switched on outside sexual activity, on a day-to-day basis. We all have the impression that if someone touches us and we don't want it, we're going to react – but it's not always the case. During an interview about writing our first book, *Jouir est un sport de combat*, Olympe told me the following anecdote. She'd gone to a local hair salon run by a guy in his mid-twenties.

'The salon is empty, it's very peaceful. After my haircut, which only takes a couple of minutes, he begins to massage my scalp, the back of my neck. It's wonderful, and I tell him so. I close my eyes and smile.

'But his hands quickly move down to my shoulder blades; his fingers massage my upper ribs. He moves over and over again to the edges of my breasts. I freeze. Is he...? I don't know what to think; I'm imagining things. He's nice and gentle, this guy. He surely can't be up to anything. After all, I'm wearing a baggy jumper, and my breasts aren't exactly fulsome... Perhaps he hadn't realised he was touching my breasts? I move in such a way as to indicate that his movements are making me uncomfortable.

He'll understand. And, indeed, his hands move back up to my shoulder blades. He talks about his fiancée – I feel paranoid.

'And then off he goes again. My brain is buzzing. I breathe in, I catch his eye in the mirror, I bore into his eyes. I ask him about his fiancée. He doesn't flinch, and continues the massage. His hands move over my torso, my belly, and glide down under the belt of my jeans. I am incapable of stopping him, of interrupting the massage. I'm scared I've got the wrong end of the stick; I'm afraid of accusing him unfairly. After all, I've just told him I liked the massage.'

> It's what we're taught from a very young age: be discreet, be attentive to what the man is saying, and go with it.

As she tells this story, Olympe expresses her anger at not being 'capable' of indicating her own limits. And I understand her: you might think that as an expert in topics concerning women's bodies (her pornographic creations, reading, daily musings), she would be all the more at ease in expressing what's good for her and what isn't. But that's simply not the case. And I'm not trying to come across as a senior lecturer in self-control: on a regular basis, and notwithstanding my own daily reflections on the subject, I too have to steer a course through my own grey areas.

In Olympe's tale, there is a broader question than the body's own limits: a female-specific difficulty in putting our own needs first. It's what we're taught from a very young age: be discreet, be attentive to what the man is saying, and go with it. Get on with playing second fiddle.

I remember being riveted by a discussion between two daughters of friends of mine. The girls, who were still at primary school, were complaining about boys. Boys, they said, took up 'all the room', ran around in the playground without thinking about others, appropriated the greater part of the space with no consideration whatsoever for any girl or boy who wasn't one of their gang. But, hey, 'They're *boys*,' one of the mothers had replied, implying that boys can't help taking up all the available space; and that girls can't help leaving them all the available space.

Olympe, dealing with her aggressive hairdresser, initially thinks she's imagining the whole thing; she finds all sorts of excuses for him, and her own discomfort moves into second place. Just like the little girls in the school playground, she was brought up (*we* were brought up) to give men priority. They make their choices in life, they place their hands on us. They say, 'Come here, I'm feeling horny!'

Where I give my consent

Olympe is listening to me. It's not the first time I've trotted out my thoughts on the importance of words, something she has also discussed, especially on her blog. And then she turns her pretty eyes on me:

> Do you feel like going to a Misungui workshop? She's an expert in talking about sex...

> Yes, yes, of course, I reply. I try to sound enthusiastic. In truth, I'm disconcerted. I, too, have areas where I'm uncomfortable: I'm a lot more at ease when surrounded by books or when talking about something I've prepared in advance than when it's a question of discussing my sexuality with strangers in a small group. But I say yes – I *consent*. Writing this book provides the opportunity to be a little adventurous – and it's not as though I'm about to spend forty-eight hours locked in a tower with hooded strangers!

Misungui is a performer, dominatrix and sexual educator. Most of all, she is very politically committed, and in particular stands up for the autonomy of the individual. The workshop takes place in her flat, which has great views over the city and the eastern suburbs of Paris. Sitting next to me and Olympe are a dozen other people, women as well as 'accompanying' men, seated on cushions and assorted material. Misungui introduces the workshop: we're going to talk about squirting, 'something that's also clumsily called female ejaculation'. It's not a topic that particularly interests me, but Olympe and I wanted to hear Misungui 'tell it how it is'.

Therefore, we seized the opportunity to take up the last two remaining spaces for this workshop.

Misungui begins by introducing herself. Her commitment as a performer, her explorations 'of sexuality, reserve and perversity'. From the outset, her words are precise and meaningful, raining down somewhat severely when she touches on feminist issues. Each one of us is then invited to take the floor to explain their motivation for participating in the workshop. Beforehand, Misungui has introduced me and Olympe; she has also asked each participant for their agreement to our taking part within the scope of writing this book. Moreover, there is no question of us abusing our position. Olympe and I are asked, as are the others, to say a few words about our feelings on squirting.

Throughout the workshop, Misungui is bent on putting her topic into words – which is exactly what is needed to pass on information, of course – but also on calling upon and listening to the words of each person present. Her vocabulary, although very precise when delving into detail, doesn't exclude plain speaking that chimes with our own realities. So we are using words like 'pussy', 'moistness', 'piss' alongside 'vaginal vestibule', 'Skene's glands' and 'clitoral hood'. We are constantly moving to and fro between expert terminology and everyday language.

I expected some embarrassment on the part of the participants, says Olympe after the workshop. But what I saw was more like shyness. Especially at the beginning.

Misungui amazed me with the precision of her explanations, I say. Was it the same for you?

Her precision – and appropriateness! She can, in the same sentence, say, 'I was horny as a bitch on heat' and 'I didn't know it, but my genitals were becoming aroused, inducing additional vaginal secretions, even though I wasn't remotely in the mood for sexual intercourse.'

We laugh. Then I think back to the person who found it so difficult to say 'my vulva', they turned puce in the face.

I thought the specific vocabulary put people ill at ease.

Hardly surprising, Olympe confirms. We are taught words like fanny or foof as a child. When you reach adulthood: nothing! So it's hard to talk about our genitals...

And to talk about sex.

That's what I took away from Misungui's workshop. Learning to correctly name the different parts of our anatomy is an essential first step.

I agree.

What's more, I say, her idea about practical exercises, while straightforward, is incredibly interesting: looking at your vulva in a mirror and naming the parts, in an auto-erotic context or not. That way, when you find yourself telling a partner you don't want this or you'd prefer that, the words come more easily.

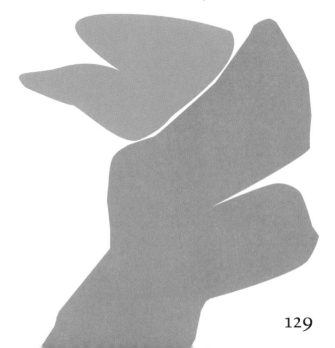

Our words, our roles

We wait until we find ourselves in an amenable place – in this instance, back at Olympe's – to pick up the conversation once more: dirty talk, also called 'erotic' talk in a recent study that looks at words use during intercourse.[38] It's worth repeating that dirty talk is a subject that comes with a warning.

Certain 'classic' phrases ('Do you like that, little bitch?', 'You're a nasty slut,' 'Fuck me hard,' etc.) that are particularly heard in mainstream porn videos are regularly called out by some feminists on the grounds that they express a patriarchal domination within one's intimate sphere – which is correct. We want to discuss that.

> Friends confided in me that they enjoyed role playing in particular moments, Olympe challenges me. If they derive pleasure from playing using codes we've been assigned, who am I to call them out?

> I heartily agree with where Olympe is going with this.

> For me, the problem comes from the fact of giving a role to just one person, whether in society or in one's intimate sphere, I say. Can't roles in domination games, for those men and women who enjoy them, be alternated? He dominates me, I dominate him; I treat him like a bastard, he treats me like a whore...

> He will penetrate me, I will penetrate him.

> Olympe and I smile, aware of the taboo that penetration still represents for many straight men.

> Do you think we can give advice to women and men who would like to engage in dirty talk but don't dare bring it up with their partner? I ask.

> Olympe agrees.

First of all, she says, remember that dirty talk goes beyond the few insults you hear in mainstream porn. Just by expressing your desires or giving instructions, you can ramp up the temperature.

Things like 'I want to feel your fingers inside me,' 'Would you like me to suck you?'

Yes. And it can start via texts, gradually: 'Thinking of you, remembering last time when, and so on.' You set the tone. Your partner will pick up on the vibe – or not, if it's not their thing.

And if it goes wrong? If a word is out of place, if a lapse creates a feeling of unease?

Well, you can't cook an omelette without breaking eggs, says Olympe. The best thing is to say the words to yourself, to tell yourself what you want to hear. Don't just try to adopt expressions heard in mainstream porn. Dirty talk does not amount to insults or domination.

I smile.

We come back to the same thing nevertheless, I say. Leave clichés behind; live your experiences to the full.

And if you fall flat on your face, if you feel you've said something that's been taken the wrong way? As for other situations like that, the best thing is to talk about it after intercourse.

That's right, I say, nodding. Talking about the sexual experience, 'debriefing' in a way, that's really important, isn't it? 'I loved what you did there,' or 'I didn't feel fully at ease at that point, and I didn't manage to say so.' It allows you to understand the other person better.

Misungui Bordelle

Communication is a *sine qua non* of my BDSM work

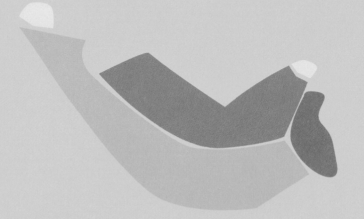

Misungui Bordelle is a committed woman. In her quest for individual autonomy and equality, she explores alternative lifestyles, including sex work. Hardly surprising, therefore, that her activities are built around words, what is said. To enable us to reflect on our own vanilla sex, we went to talk to Misungui about the safe working practices she has put in place as a professional.

Olympe de Gê (O de G)   As a sex worker, you earn your living as a dominatrix ...

Misungui Bordelle (MB)   Yes, though I do plenty of other things, too. I also take part in erotic podcasts, I perform in feminist porn films and I offer sex education workshops. As a dominatrix I specialise in shibari, which is the Japanese art of rope bondage between consenting individuals.

O d G   Do you talk much while you work?

MB   Communication is the *sine qua non* of this type of activity. But that certainly doesn't mean I'm asking my rope bunny every other minute if things are OK. We agree a framework in advance so as to enter into the spirit of the activity as calmly as possible, both for the runner and the bunny. It allows the rope bunny to fully let go while ensuring the dominatrix remains vigilant and empathetic.

Stéphanie Estournet (SE)   Let's suppose I contact you because I'm interested in being tied up. What happens? Do we meet?

MB   Woah! Hold your horses! First you'd receive a standard email in which I broadly outline what it is I do. That enables me to eliminate some of the requests I don't want to take up. For example, I don't dress in typical leather or latex dominatrix clothes. If you want to see me with that in mind, then it's no.

SE   What happens next if I am still enthusiastic about what you're proposing ...

MB   If you don't have any experience, you'll receive another email detailing how a session is run and setting out what happens during that first meeting. For example, I explain that it's better there's no genital contact.

SE   Why?

MB   During an initial session you might be knocked sideways by what you experience and find yourself in an altered state of consciousness. As a result you might want to have genital contact but subsequently regret it.

That's why I prefer to wait until people are more seasoned before agreeing to satisfy their request for genital contact.

O de G   How do you work out the communication you mentioned?

MB   At the beginning of the first session I explain the physical risks involved as well as my way of communicating, in particular using safe language – simple, agreed words that allow the people I've tied up with rope to let me know how they are feeling: green, everything is fine; orange, things are hotting up; red, untie me. I check we understand each other.

SE   What happens next?

MB   I do a simple shibari bondage tie-up that lasts about twenty minutes. We have a break and a debrief. Then we start the second tie-up that lasts between forty-five minutes and an hour and a quarter, depending on the person's mood and state of mind. From then on, I can generally see things clearly: I understand them better, I can gauge their limits.

OdG   Why 'generally'?

MB   Some people find it really difficult to say what they are feeling. In that case I might suggest asking them during the session: 'Everything OK?' But from the outset some individuals say they are incapable of even replying to that simple query. So I may decide not to tie them up.

It's a game for two: the individual needs to trust me but I also need to be able to trust them. When you're doing extreme things, you risk putting yourself in danger if you are unable to judge exactly where you are at.

O de G   I think those of us enjoying conventional sex can learn something from that – even if we're not encountering the same risks. A simple example: if when it crops up, I'm not sure whether I want to be penetrated, then I need to be aware of it and say 'No, I don't want to.' Any doubts should push us to protect ourselves rather than accept an activity we're not sure we want.

MB   Saying 'Yes, I want to do that' or 'No, I don't fancy that' allows those involved to know exactly where they stand. Non-verbal utterances like groans, cries and even tears can have all sorts of explanations. Maybe you're crying because you feel bad - but then again it might be because you're experiencing a powerful sensation of letting go. Only you know. If you don't communicate it to me, my interpretation may be very wide off the mark. And there's a risk I might react in a way that could be inappropriate.

SE   Which implies the need to be connected to what you're feeling and to be able to be specific.

MB   If all you tell me is, 'I'm not OK,' then I don't know what to do to help you: release a toe that's got caught? Take you in my arms? Completely untie you? It's essential any communication is crystal clear. But where grey areas remain then if in doubt I will untie you.

SE   At the end of the day only I know what's good for me ...

O d G You have to learn how to express yourself until it becomes an integral part of you. Consent involves a whole series of mechanisms that should form an integral part of any relationship.

MB   I practise BDSM, an approach to sexuality that is neither less nor more intense than conventional sex. Sharing your intimacy means accepting to show your vulnerable side. In all relationships there is an element of risk. You have to accept it.

At the same time there is a notion of responsibility that does not allow any shortcuts. On this, men have a great deal to learn, especially when it involves listening to women and accepting what they are saying. It's high time they left more space for women to express themselves – or they could even create this space themselves and perhaps ask women clear and direct questions and listen carefully to their answers.

SE   Do you have any reading recommendations?

MB   One of my bibles for gender studies when I was at university was *Thinking Sex: Notes for a Radical Theory of the Politics of Sexuality* by Gayle Rubin - that includes, in passing, a nice reference to Michel Foucault.

It's a little hard-going in the sense that you need to be used to reading university essays but it's a gold mine as far as gender, sex and feminism are concerned. There is also a whole chapter on a sociological survey carried out by lesbians who practise BDSM. Fascinating.

Another classic that's far more accessible is *The Ethical Slut* by Dossie Easton and Janet W. Hardy which looks at polyamory, consent and questions concerning communication. It's stuffed with practical advice and concrete examples which make it straightforward to read and the information easy to grasp.

On polyamory, consent and in particular the notion of enthusiastic consent, I really enjoy the blog *Les fesses de la crémière* (www.lesfess esdelacremiere.wordpress.com). It's written by a man, it's full of insights and provides masses of references.

Finally, on lessons in shibari, conferences and online performances with a feminist and inclusive twist that drills down into the issue of consent, I recommend *Shibari Study* (www.shibaristudy.com). It's a really fabulous English-language site containing information that is both free to watch and subscription only.

---

38 Superdrug Online Doctirs, 2020. 990 European and American (from 18 to 83 years old) respondents about their sexual talk .https://onlinedoctor.superdrug.com/pillow-talk/#

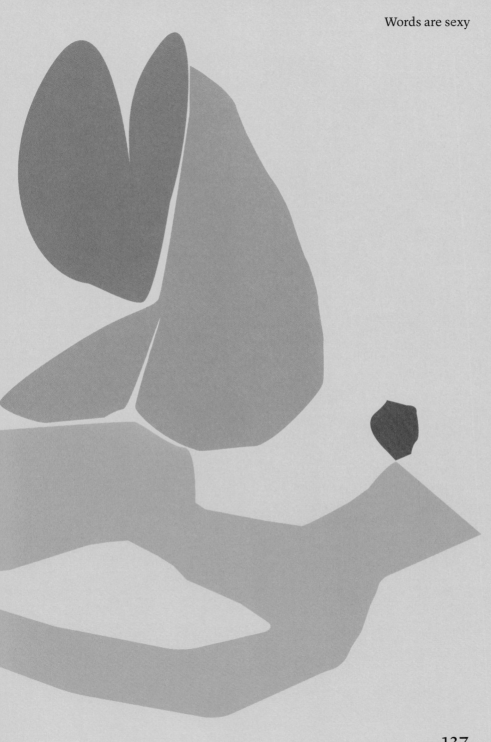

Chapter 8

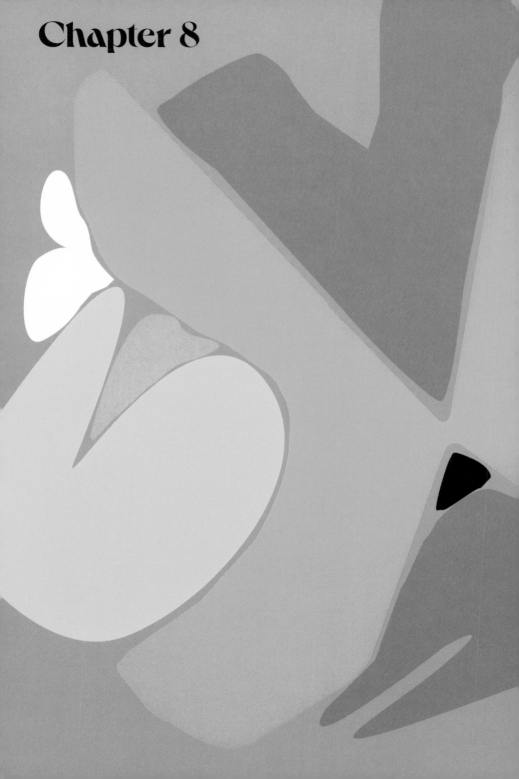

Name the pain and treat it

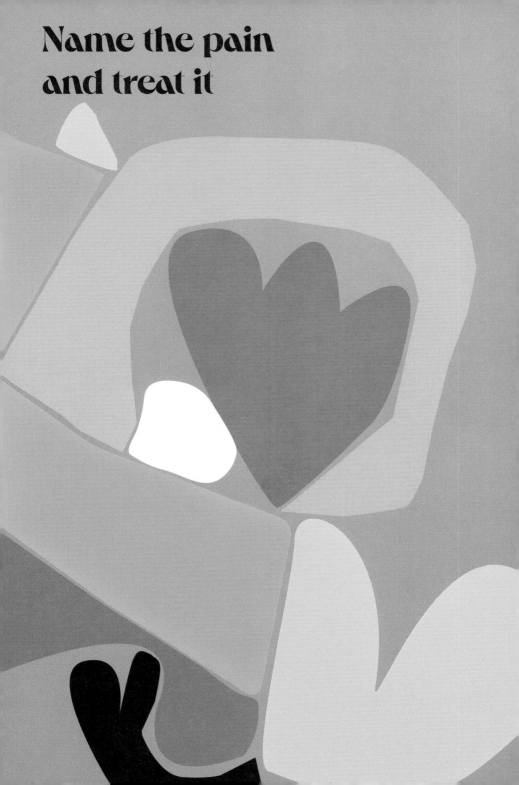

Tuesday 22 February 2022

I've been invited to go to the cinema this evening. There will be a showing of the documentary *Female Pleasure* on a small screen in the Latin quarter, and I've been invited to say a few words at the end. I readily accepted. I like this film, and find it asks many essential questions. Why, all around the world and stretching back millennia, do men attack women's bodies? Why is there this universal need to control female sexuality?

In *Female Pleasure*, the director, Barbara Miller, introduces us to five women activists. Hailing from very different countries and cultures, all five suffered violent, patriarchal oppression – because they are women – that has affected their gender, their sexuality, their right to self-determination. These women each fight in their own way to take back control over their bodies and their freedom.

▶ In Germany, Doris Wagner, a former nun, left the Catholic Church following incidents of rape and sexual attack at the hands of two priests. The facts were hushed up by the Mother Superior. Since then, she's fought to make the Church acknowledge these crimes and abuses of power.

▶ In the United States, Deborah Feldman was forced into marriage aged seventeen.[39] She fled the oppression of her Hasidic community in Brooklyn with her baby, and built herself a new life in Europe, far from the anger and threats of her former family members.

▶ The Japanese fine-art artist, Rokudenashiko, was arrested in 2014 and risks two years' imprisonment for having produced and exhibited a 3-D model of her vulva. The representation of her genitals, with the aim of reverse-demonising the female body and its representations, was ironically viewed as 'obscene' in the country of the *Kanamara matsuri* – a festival that, each spring, exhibits thousands of phalluses in every part of the mega-city of Kawasaki. To avoid prison, Rokudenashiko was forced into exile.

▶ Like too many other Indian women, Vithika Yadav suffered aggression and harassment. The first woman in her family to escape an arranged marriage, she wed the man she loved and set up the website Love Matters,[40] which talks about sex and love in a country where 'the concept of love doesn't exist,' and where sexual violence is on the rise.

> Born in a Muslim Somali family, the Londoner Leyla Hussein was excised at age seven, hemmed in and held down by the women in her family. Since her own daughter's birth, she has been fighting against female genital mutilation (FGM). 'Touching or cutting the genital areas of any child constitutes a sexual offence,' she says. 'We have to call a spade a spade.' Her determination and charisma sear the mind, as do the giant vulvas in plasticine that she butchers with enormous secateurs to illustrate the different variants of mutilation. She wages her fierce campaign to safeguard the physical integrity and sexual self-determination of women in the United Kingdom as well as in Africa. In London, she brings awareness of the issue to young Muslim men and organises support groups for female victims; in Kenya, she campaigns in Maasai villages against this practice that 'has no cultural basis'. FGM, she says, is neither an African nor an Asian problem. It is, first and foremost, a 'global problem'.

These five narratives have affected me to such an extent that I remember *Female Pleasure* as though I saw it yesterday, but it came out in 2018. It's probably because the stories of these five women talk about physical oppression, here and now – a topic that is still, and constantly, relevant. They relate the pain inflicted on our bodies and on our women's genitals: a subject that affects us all in our very flesh.

Major political stakes

Everywhere in the world, in every culture and every religious context, women are physically dominated by men through pain and humiliation. The film *Female Pleasure* drills down to ask why; the anthropologist, Françoise Héritier, who died in 2017, had an answer. According to her, universal masculine domination can be explained by the need for men to take control of something they are physically unable to do: reproduction. 'Since men cannot bear children using their own bodies, whereas women give birth to girls and boys, they have arranged things so that female bodies are at their disposal,' she said in 2016.

Our bodies, our genitals and our women's sexualities are major political issues. The oppression we suffer on the part of patriarchal societies wanting to hold on to this control is violent. But while this violence is often physical, it can also be symbolic and take the form of insidious psychological manipulation. In their book *Anatomy of Oppression*, the two FEMEN activists

Inna Shevchenko and Pauline Hillier explain how women are educated from an early age to see their genitals as a source of humiliation: 'Vagina shaming works in the name of moral tradition and reinforces religious arguments. While still very young, little girls are persuaded that their vulva is dirty, that they shouldn't touch it, [should] never mention it and [should] only ever show it to their future spouse.'

The sad consequences of this systemic denigration is a total ignorance on the part of young girls of their bodies. Harried by taboos, bans and shame, women do not know what their own vulvas look like, since they daren't look at or touch them. A study in France in 2017 revealed that 35 per cent of female respondents had never seen their own clitoris – and 20 per cent didn't know where it was located.[41] These figures astonished the media... but not me. And I know only too well why: I myself was ignorant about my own sexual anatomy for years. Until I was nineteen, I thought urine passed out through the clitoris! Given the clitoris somewhat resembles a small penis, it seemed normal to me that, like for boys, bodily fluids streamed out of this appendage...

Shevchenko and Hillier explain that women experience actual mental suppression of their genitals: 'By hearing it described as a source of impurity and shame, they have annihilated it, switched it off, turned it into a chained-up wild animal cowering in the far corner of its cage that should only be released if the leash is handed over to a husband-master.'

Some feminists call this phenomenon mental excision: the Egyptian writer and feminist, Nawal El Saadawi, known as the 'Simone de Beauvoir of the Arab world' and excised as a child, used to refer to 'the mental excision' of Western women.

In reality, if mothers perpetuate this tradition of having their little girls excised, it's through fear their daughters won't otherwise find a husband. Remaining unmarried seems to them worse than suffering FGM. One can find a similar rhetoric in France, the UK and the USA, where content and advertisements directed towards women, speak of little else other than this fear of having to live without a man. A 'sad fate' that may conveniently be avoided by frantically consuming cosmetics, fashion, sport, etc., etc. ... all while remaining ignorant of our own anatomy. I think it's far more urgent for us to re-appropriate our women's bodies. To observe them, listen to them, learn to understand them. To move away from the shame foisted upon us as far as our bodies are concerned. I believe we urgently need to know how our bodies work, how to scrutinise our pain and listen to it. To remember that being a woman does not condemn us to suffering. That it is essential to take care of ourselves as only we know how.

7.30pm

The screening is taking place in a couple of hours. I jot down a few notes in my phone. On the stage with me and chairing the event is an African-European author and podcaster, Axelle Jah Njiké, who is active in the battle against FGM and part of the GAMS Federation (Group for the Abolition of Forced Marriages and other Traditional Practices that Harm Women's and Children's Health). I read one of her articles in *Le Monde*, and her words resonate powerfully with those of Leyla Hussein as she talks about FGM as a 'global problem':

> Excision is nothing to do with race, colour or religion. It's nothing other than mutilation. Inflicted on women because of their sex.
> It is practised in Africa, Asia, the Middle East, India and in Indonesia for the same reason: the opprobrium with which women's sexuality, and more particularly their pleasure, has been regarded since the dawn of time. The clitoris has nothing to do with reproduction and therefore is considered useless.[42]

Useless, and apparently shameful. Even dangerous. Could it be that the pleasure the clitoris offers represents a source of emancipation that could threaten the patriarchy? Today, across the globe, 200 million women have suffered some form of FGM. Three million little girls each year risk being subjected to it. Every eleven seconds, FGM is carried out on a girl child.[43] Although these customs are historically more widespread across the African continent, they can be found in every region of the world, including European countries with immigrant populations. Thus, in Europe, it is estimated that 500,000 adult women have suffered a form of FGM.

What can one say against excision?

Despite the horror these figures cause me, I have preferred to keep quiet when others talk about excision. As a white woman, I fear exhibiting racism despite myself in discussing practices that are widespread in Black societies in particular. Would it not smack of neo-colonialism to denounce the barbarity of others, rather than concentrating on the aggressions inflicted on women under my very own eyes? Wouldn't I do better to take a look at what's happening in my own backyard?

Axelle's words reassure me: 'FGM is not a "White" or "Black" woman's issue. It's every woman's issue. Whether we've suffered the brutality of the knife or not. It is a reminder that we have to campaign for women to have power and sovereignty, the right to exercise free choice and re-establish their original free will, dignity and sexuality. It's all part of our universal right to have freedom in our bodies, to draw strength from our sexual potential and affirm our claim to be autonomous citizens.'

It is uncomfortable to talk about FGM, given that my body has never known this suffering, nor have I experienced the betrayal by one's nearest and dearest that FGM represents. I can rely only on what I've read, the words of Leyla Hussein in *Female Pleasure*, for example, to try to understand. There is, however, one thing of which I am convinced: FGM is one of a multitude of violent actions inflicted on women by men in order to keep them under a yoke. 'The patriarchal society is at the root of excision,' Leyla Hussein confirms.[44]

Force and power

'Excision signifies female strength that has been crushed, dominated, muzzled. It illustrates just how long, throughout history, we have been the ones who always seem to be the losers, sexually speaking, those who submit to sex. This way of doing things must change.' With these words, Axelle Jah Njiké opens our discussion in front of the audience who have come to watch *Female Pleasure*.

I take the floor. I won't speak further about pain; these women have all done so with great force and power. I will, instead, talk about what comes after the pain: the caring. I want to tell the women seated on the Accattone cinema velvet chairs, the young girl chewing gum next to her mother, the lady sitting in the front row with her chic silver perm, that our bodies are ours, our sex organs are ours.

No one will take care of them in our steads, for the simple reason that no one can do so. No God, no moral compass, no doctor, no spiritual authority, no philosophy, no man, no relative, is able to know better than we do what is good for us and our own bodies.

It's up to us to reconnect with our bodies; it's up to us to bring our genitals out of their cages. It's up to us to pay attention to our pains and pleasures. It's our bodies that we need to learn to listen to, and listen to well, before we listen to anything directed at us from others.

Labiaplasty, really?

I'm walking through the Latin Quarter. The winter evening breeze blushes my cheeks. I'm returning home on foot, and I know that when I get into bed, my body will be grateful for this hour's walk.

As I pass through the streets, the adrenaline accumulated while speaking in public subsides. Tiredness drops away from my spine, the back of my head. My forehead, my eyebrows relax. My brain even seems to soften... After the intense concentration of being in front of an audience, it feels like break time: a thousand thoughts come flooding into my brain. I can't banish Leyla Hussein's account of her life from my mind. I realise I didn't, in the end, even mention the words 'mutilation' or 'excision' during this evening's discussion. That old, familiar sense of unease overcomes me once again. And yet... As a white woman, there is one topic in particular that taxes me more directly: labiaplasty, another form of mutilation of a woman's genitals, and in great demand in the West.

An aesthetically 'perfect' vulva – to what end?

Labiaplasty is a surgical operation to reduce the volume of the inner lips of the vulva. While an aesthetic intervention is in no way comparable to a sexual attack undertaken by force using a knife on a young girl, the issue still deserves examination. Labiaplasty is only recommended on medical grounds in extremely rare instances, when the length of the internal lips interferes with comfort or causes pain: when doing sport, for example, or during sexual intercourse. Yet requests for labiaplasty operations have significantly increased over the last few years, despite the high costs involved.[45] In France, 4,600 women opted for the procedure in 2016, compared to 1,839 in 2010.[46] The American Society for Aesthetic Plastic Surgery (ASAPS) recently released its national cosmetic surgery statistics for 2016. One statistic in particular stood out to me: labiaplasty procedures increased by over 23% last year, making it the second fastest growing procedure for 2016. According to surgeons, patients requesting this operation tend to be very young: they are chiefly between eighteen and twenty-two years of age, although some are under eighteen; in the United Kingdom, no fewer than 156 girls aged under eighteen had labiaplasty procedures in 2015. In the main, they had one thing in common: their vulva was a normal size, and their motivation was not based on medical grounds (pain, embarrassment) but on aesthetic grounds. They want their epilated vulva to be perfectly shaped and not prominent when wearing leggings or other figure-hugging clothes.

The inner lips contain a large number of nerve endings; they are involved in sexual pleasure. Labiaplasty, like any surgical operation, is not an anodyne option. For years, the Californian activist Jessica Pin has been warning patients and the medical profession about the dangers of this procedure, which is still far too inadequately regulated.

Aged eighteen, Jessica believed her inner lips were excessively long and thought her vulva was abnormal. Wanting the intimate parts of her body to conform to a certain standard of beauty, she went down the route of labiaplasty. The consent form for surgery stated 'excision of excessive lip volume'. But instead of that, the surgeon cut off all her inner lips and reduced the size of her clitoral hood, something she had not requested. After the operation, when she touched her vulva, there was no longer any sensation whatsoever. The dorsal nerves of her clitoris had been inadvertently sectioned during the procedure. Since then, she has been unable to reach orgasm.

The consequences on Jessica Pin's mental health have been devastating. After years of depression, she asked herself what might have caused this medical error. Suspecting a poor understanding of the anatomy of the vulva, she discovered that the sexual function of the inner lips is rarely described in medical literature, and the distal pathway of the dorsal nerves of the clitoris did not even feature in the anatomical diagrams found in gynaecological textbooks! Since then, Jessica has participated in vulval dissections and co-published a study of the anatomy of the clitoris.[47] She has contacted more than twenty textbook publishers; five of them have updated their publications with a correct anatomical description of the clitoris.

The growing popularity of labiaplasty is nothing other than an indicator of the exhortations visited on women to have a body designed to please men. What's more, this operation has been nicknamed 'getting a designer vagina'. An expression that, in itself, sums up the ignorance in which we live as soon as we get down to talking about female anatomy: labiaplasty has nothing to do with the vagina, which is an internal organ that acts as a conduit. This ignorance of the anatomy of the clitoris is widespread, even among healthcare professionals officially qualified to use a scalpel on a vulva. And it can wreak havoc. In the United States, it is estimated that over 1,000 female patients are mutilated by surgeons this way each year.[48]

Sadly, I get the impression the clitoris isn't really safe anywhere.

Night

As soon as I'm in bed, I feel myself dropping off to sleep. As predicted, the walk prepared me for slumber. Tomorrow, I'm meeting Stéphanie straight after a medical appointment; I'm going to get an IUD fitted. It's something that can be a bit painful; the memory of the pinching sensation when the last one was inserted still makes me wince. But this time, it won't be that bossy female gynae who'll do it but my family doctor. He's my age, and not someone who believes his ten years of study entitle him to know more than I do about what I'm feeling or what my needs are. He's there to listen, he asks questions, he pays attention to my answers. I really appreciate his lateral thinking, offering considerate and gentle care.

Wednesday 23 February 2022

The IUD fitting goes well, and I leave my doctor's surgery with a smile on my face. However nervous I feel when I step inside this place, I always feel better afterwards. I thank him for that; I'm not asking for much, but the way one is treated is a powerful and important factor! I feel totally at ease talking to him, and I know that any physical examination will be carried out delicately, painlessly. That fills me with confidence. At the slightest concern, I wouldn't think twice about telling him.

The 'weaker sex' – such nonsense...

From a clinical perspective, the women who turn up at doctors' surgeries are often more vulnerable than men. This is, of course, not down to their biology (the idea of the 'weaker sex' is pure nonsense), but to psycho-social factors: their status or their family and economic situations, which are more likely to be on a knife-edge. Women are also at greater risk of violence and sexual assault. In order to offer proper treatment, healthcare professionals could, for example, be trained in systematically screening for signs of violence, and could learn to build a rapport where patient and doctor feel they are on an equal footing (as my doctor does), rather than one of experts ruling over their patients, as is all too often the case.

Beyond discrimination, there is also a high incidence of traumatic, gender-based violence. When the hashtag #payetongyneco (a #metoo movement in the gynaecologist field) burst on to the French social media scene, I spent hours reading women's accounts of the gynaecological and obstetric violations they had suffered. The situations described were mindlessly sexist; but what struck me most forcefully were the accounts of medical deeds enacted without the patient's consent – 'When you jump because of an invasive (unannounced) gesture and you're told: you're not supposed to enjoy it' – or without showing the patient any respect – 'Oh, for heaven's sake, it's only two fingers…' I also read about women recounting feelings of having been raped during a clinical examination, or even during childbirth, because the medical interventions were violent and/or not consented to.

As a film director and producer of porn films in particular, I have to deal with the question of consent when filming intimate scenes: how do I ensure an actor doesn't feel pressured? How can I be certain she or he doesn't do anything they don't want to, or put up with anything they don't want to happen? How can I be sure the touch of unknown hands on their body is an OK experience? How can I ensure they always feel able to ask if they want a gesture, contact or scene to stop? While filming *Une dernière fois*, I used a range of actions to manage and safeguard as far as possible the consent of the actors. Several weeks before filming, we agreed on the sex acts, giving as much detail as possible. We used questionnaires, asking things like: using saliva as a lubricant, is that OK or not? Your saliva? The other person's?

Porn and the gynaecologist: something in common!

Through reading so many accounts of gynaecological and obstetric violations, I realised something: making a porn film and going to see your gynaecologist share something important. In both instances, you have, on the one hand, a person who exposes their genitalia in an unfamiliar environment, and, on the other, one or more fully dressed participants surrounding them and dictating what and how things happen. In both cases, it's a fundamentally asymmetrical situation. And the fact it involves someone's genitals, their sexuality, makes it all the more sensitive. Something tells me that if in the world of porn it's possible to reflect on the notion of consent and work actively around it, doctors and gynaecologists could do the same!

And what's more, there's no harm in letting them know: women have been protesting against medical mistreatment for 'only' fifty years! In the 1970s, American feminists were already denouncing violent paternalism on the part of gynaecologists, to the point where a medical resistance movement was formed: women began re-appropriating their bodies and their vulvas. A bible on issues of health, care and knowledge of the female body, *Our Bodies, Ourselves* was published in 1969. In its wake, self-help gynaecological workshops were set up, in which women collectively practised self-examination: they were the ones inserting a speculum into their vaginas and checking – or admiring! – their cervices with a mirror.

Long live young health professionals!

3.15pm

After leaving the doctor's surgery, I meet up with Stéphanie and we walk aimlessly, chatting away. Spring is on its way, the warmth of the sun is much appreciated. Stéphanie talks about the violence she has suffered as a woman, especially around childbirth (she has two daughters).

> We often talk about this in connection with male or older male and female doctors. If I look back at my experience, the violations came from various quarters: from the medical technician inserting an endo-vaginal probe as though he was about to rip open my belly, to the female obstetrician asking me wasn't I ashamed to have put on so much weight.

It's not the first time I've heard Stéphanie adopt a fatalistic tone when talking about these issues.

We're making progress, word is spreading, she says, but not
so long ago, women had no choice other than to grit their teeth.
Menstrual pain, psychological distress linked to motherhood,
an abortion, or even having an IUD inserted, like you've
just had... We were expected to accept procedures in silence.

In good moments, I'm glad to think that we are putting that period
behind us.

It's what I told myself the day I came out of a medical practice
dedicated to women, run by young healthcare professionals,
Stéphanie continues, smiling. Before each step, the gynaecologist
and afterwards the radiographer would explain the examination,
asking me for permission to touch such-and-such a place. I could
hardly believe it. 'Why are these women asking me when they are
entitled to do anything?' It was only sometime later that I realised
that no, a healthcare professional is not someone with authority,
they are not entitled to do anything. You don't hand your body over
to them as if you're leaving your car in the garage!

8.20pm

Following on from what Stéphanie was saying, I'd like people to stop thinking
it's normal for a woman to suffer. That you just have to put up with it, hold
your head up high. Sometimes you simply can't, and we should feel able
to say 'I'm in pain' and to take a break when their bodies are suffering
(periods, menopause, etc.). We need a global acceptance of something along
the lines of the period pause that exists in South Korea, Japan and Indonesia,
and will soon come into effect in Spain. Self-care, comfort and well-being are
not threatening concepts, even in a world bent on corporate productivism.
And taking care of yourself, as a knock-on effect, means taking care of others...

More and more health professionals – doctors, but also midwives,
alternative carers, etc. – work by listening to their patients. Perhaps we
should start by asking them first and foremost.

24 June 2022

So much time has passed. Stéphanie and I, very busy, have put our project on hold. But here is some edifying news that brings us back to it. A real cold shower! The United States Supreme Court overturned Roe v Wade. Individual states are now able to choose whether to ban, limit or grant the right to an abortion. We knew it would come to this: the alarm bells started ringing years ago. And some states made sure they were ready for 'the big day', swiftly banning terminations of pregnancy beyond six weeks – in some cases, even where there is evidence of rape and/or incest. In my head, I hear Simone de Beauvoir's 1974 warning a couple of months before French deputies put the Veil Law, authorising abortion, to the vote: 'Don't forget that it will only take a political, economic or religious crisis for women's rights to be questioned once more. These rights are never enshrined in perpetuity.'

In the most influential democracy in the world, women are gradually being denied their rights to choose what they wish for their bodies.

I think about all those individuals who are pregnant today who do not want the pregnancy but are doomed to give birth, to care for and educate a child, and so on. I think about those people who risk legal ramifications following a miscarriage... What is being said about the men who got them pregnant? Do they, too, have obligations? Are they going to take care of these individuals during their pregnancies, commit to contributing to, caring for and educating the children? If they fail to do so, will they, in turn, risk fines and maybe prison?

Let's stand up and defend our rights!

In France in April 1971, 343 women signatories (including the actress Delphine Seyrig, the film director Agnès Varda, the lawyer Gisèle Halimi and the writers Simone de Beauvoir and Françoise Sagan) of Manifesto 343 declared in the *Nouvel Observateur* magazine that they had all had a backstreet abortion, and demanded the right to legal terminations of pregnancy. Four years later, the Veil Law granted their request. 'I constructed myself around these stories of struggle, of women who bear witness, reflect, speak out, unite,' Stéphanie told me one day, recalling former journalist colleagues who reported on the Bobigny trial[49] or on the MLF demonstrations.[50]

Today, in solidarity with all women governed by legislation banning them access to abortions, we could echo the gesture expressed by our older sisters. In our manifesto, we could affirm that no one has the right to decide on our behalf what we do with our bodies. Voluntary termination of a pregnancy should be a right for anyone, and someone's choice to have an abortion should not be up for discussion). We could emphasise that banning the right to abortion has in no measure reduced recourse to abortion. A woman who does not want to have a child will do everything in her power to end the pregnancy, even at a cost to her life. Approximately 25 million risky backstreet abortions are carried out every year around the world.[51]

The fight against the mutilation of women, and the fights for the right to abortion, the right to healthcare... So many areas that indicate just how far our bodies represent a realm to be defended, to be cherished, over which we must keep watch. This discussion with Stéphanie motivates me to seek out caring professionals and healthcare providers for myself and for the women in my life. Lists of safe professionals are recommended by patients and include non-sexist gynaecologists,[52] non-fat-shaming doctors,[53] LGBTQIA+-friendly male and female carers[54] and Black healthcare professionals. I would also like to move away from a hyper-medicalised approach in favour of listening, exchanging ideas and sharing experiences. Whether we're talking about political decisions, our intimate body parts or another medical context, we should be mistresses of our own bodies in every instance.

> So many areas that indicate just how far our bodies represent a realm to be defended, to cherish, over which we must keep watch.

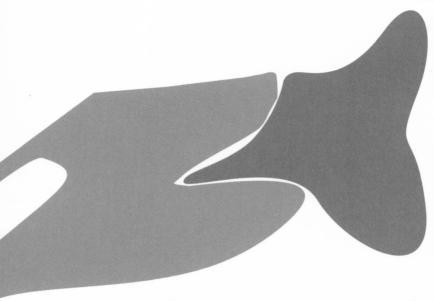

39 Deborah Feldman is the author of *Unorthodox: The Scandalous Rejection of My Hasidic Roots*, Simon & Schuster, 2012. It was adapted into a Netflix series in 2020, directed by Maria Schrader.

40 https://lovematters.in.

41 Study carried out by the Terpan Laboratory on a group of 580 women (18-25 years old), 2017.

42 In this article, Axelle Jah Njiké retraces the fight that led to the official reporting of female genital mutilations, and their criminalisation: '*L'Afrique intime. Femme noire, femme blanche, ensemble contre l'excision*', *Le Monde*, 19 July 2016.

43 'Leyla Hussein: The Cruel Cut', Oslo Freedom Forum, YouTube, 14 June 2017 (https://www.youtube.com/watch?v=rBV1zKft3oY).

44 In BEH (Weekly Epidemiological Bulletin), Santé publique France (https://www.letemps.ch/societe/leyla-hussein-societe-patriarcale-racine-lexcision).

45 €2000-3,000 for an operation carried out in France.

46 Figures revealed by Essity Intimate Care Survey France, relayed by Nana (https://www.stephenmchen.com/post/why-is-labiaplasty-on-the-rise).

47 Kelling, J. A., Erickson, C. R., Pin, P. G. & Pin, J. 2020, 'Anatomical Dissection of the Dorsal Nerve of the Clitoris,' *Aesthetic Surgery Journal*, vol. 40, no. 5, pp. 541–547.

48 Read about this in feminist writer Suzannah Weiss's article 'The Insidious Reasons Doctors Are Botching Labiaplasties,' *The Establishment*, 17 January 2019 (https://theestablishment.co/the-insidious-reasons-doctors-are-botching-labiaplasties/index.html).

49 In 1972, the trial of Marie-Claire Chevalier, aged sixteen, took place in Bobigny (Seine-Saint-Denis) on an indictment of illegal abortion. At the time, termination of pregnancy was banned in France. Four other women were tried for aiding and abetting. The advocacy for the defence by lawyer Gisèle Halimi was spectacularly successful; it contributed to the wake-up call and decriminalisation of abortion that came into force with the Veil Law on 17 January 1975.

50 The MLF (Women's Liberation Movement) is a feminist movement founded in 1970 with the aim of continuing the work of American Women's Lib.

51 2018 figures, Family Planning: www.planning-familial.org/sites/default/files/2019-01/2018-09-focus-avortement-Monde.pdf.

52 In France: https://gynandco.wordpress.com/trouver-un-e-soignant-e/; in French-speaking Switzerland: https://adopteunegyneco.wordpress.com; in Belgium: https://gotogyneco.be (for lesbian and bisexual women).

53 https://graspolitique.wordpress.com/liste-safe/.

54 https://www.medecin-gay-friendly.fr.

Martin Winckler

'Nobody should make choices for us about our bodies or our health'

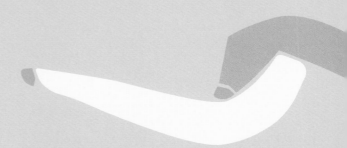

Novelist, essayist, translator, critic...
Martin Winckler, for many years,
combined his writing activities with
being a doctor, working in particular
with women (gynaecology, pregnancy
terminations) in France. Today, Winckler,
now a Canadian national, is no longer
a practising doctor. In his writings and
in public, he defends the need to turn
our backs on the authoritarian doctor-
patient relationship in order to provide
more appropriate care.

Stéphanie Estournet (SE)   Can you define care?

Martin Winckler (MW)   Caring is about listening to the person who is suffering. It's giving them advice, enabling them to understand the situation and make choices, if need be.

Olympe de Gê (O de G)   If I've understood you correctly, the role of the doctor is to be at the service of the patient?

MW   It should be that, anyway. But being a doctor means you are often viewed as having status that conveys authority – especially in countries with a Catholic tradition. The fact that the doctor is supposed to be 'the expert' seems to set up a hierarchical relationship – all the more prevalent when it involves women because it falls into a patriarchal framework.

SE   Women today do speak out about all kinds of brutal practices, some of them abusive, when their questions, their pains, are not being taken into consideration...

O de G   The family doctor who tells us, rolling his eyes, that, 'Yes, periods are painful; but there we are, it doesn't last...'

SE   'You've put on a lot of weight, Mrs X. Being pregnant doesn't mean you can do what you want with food.'

O de G   'If you sleep with anything on two legs then, of course, you're behaving in a risky fashion.'

SE   'It's time you got on with it. At your age, I already had two children.'

O de G   'If it really hurt, you'd be screaming.'

MW   So many humiliating, painful, unacceptable situations. And so much to deconstruct. Some aspects seem to be an automatic part of the ritual of consulting a doctor, whereas they urgently need to be called out. For example, examinations are not always necessary. A patient may, for reasons of their own, not want an examination; no authority should pressure the patient into doing something against their will. Another important aspect: a doctor, whether a specialist or family doctor, should not ask personal questions outside the scope of caring for their patients. In the case of gynaecologists, too many stories reveal intrusive lines of questioning.

O de G   I went to see a doctor after experiencing pain during intercourse; the doctor asked me what my preferred position was, and that of my partner. That shocked me.

MW   I understand! And while we're discussing the basic behavioural principles, a doctor shouldn't make personal comments about a patient's body, either. 'You're too fat,' 'You're lucky to have such a great bust,' and so on, are not what a doctor is saying; they reflect the individual *behind* the doctor. And we don't give a damn what this person thinks outside their purely professional domain.

SE   Certain examinations are necessary...

MW   No medical examination is necessary. It's up to each person to take care of themselves. We do what we feel is best for us. There are, however, recommendations, such as when trying to screen for a serious illness or a cancer.

O de G   So, as far as gynaecology is concerned, no smear test or breast examination every time you see the gynae?

MW   Unless you have any family history, breast examination shouldn't take place before the patient is twenty-five – unless you request it. From that age onwards, it is recommended, but not necessary – in the knowledge that most breast cancers develop in women over fifty years of age.

SE   And what about smear tests?

MW   You're recommended to get a screening smear test every three years between the ages of twenty-five and sixty-five, whatever your sexual orientation. However, it's important to remember that all women who have sexual intercourse might become infected. The papillomavirus infection can develop from contact with a phallus, and also through finger contact.

O de G   Information that should come from the gynaecologist...

MW   Or from the family doctor. There is no need to go and see a gynaecologist. Initially, youngsters don't know what route to take, who to turn to. They need to be informed that certain products, like the morning-after pill and condoms, are freely available. Information can be found at the click of a button, and there is more and more literature available that enables them to find things out. Then you can choose who you want to go and see for medical care, irrespective of your age. We should ask ourselves the question: what do we expect from a healthcare professional? To be listened to? To get advice? It's rare, for example, that patients systematically want to be examined. If my doctor's tendency to systematically examine me bothers me, then I can let them know and/or change doctors.

SE   If I'm going along to get contraception, then I have to agree to an examination...

MW   Why? A woman seeking contraception isn't ill. She's making a choice about her life. If you go to your doctor, for example, to ask for the pill, you're not caught in a trap and needing someone to help you get out; you're pre-empting falling in there in the first place, should one lie in your path – that's a whole different ball game! And there's no need to have a clinical examination – unless you request one, of course, because you are in some discomfort, or have a problem.

O de G   What's your approach to pregnancy terminations?

MW   In Quebec, where I live, abortion is legal throughout pregnancy, although clinics offering terminations after the second trimester are becoming increasingly rare, prioritising serious foetal abnormalities. In France, an abortion is not considered to be a healthcare procedure but an ideological stance: is it right or wrong to have an abortion, to terminate a pregnancy after X weeks of amenorrhea, and so forth?

It's important to remember that only persons with a uterus are in a position to choose whether or not they opt for an abortion. The genetic co-genitor does not have a say. Should the pregnant woman decide to go ahead with the pregnancy, the co-genitor runs no physical risk themselves. You can't oblige someone to go through with a pregnancy, nor can you force them to terminate it. She is mistress of her body. It's her territory.

SE   I've realised, through talking to my adolescent daughters, that we say very little about suffering. Hardly anything. It's as though we've taken on board that, as women, we're going to suffer in any case. And that's it's better to keep quiet, not make a song and dance about it.

MW   When I carried out abortions, I used to go and see the women after the procedure. To my question, 'Are you in pain?' the answer was invariably, 'It's bearable.' Using this anecdote, I agree with what you're saying: women from Catholic traditions believe that pain is part of their lives and that they are expected not to complain. The same isn't true, for example, among women from the Maghreb region of North Africa, who are much more likely to express their physical suffering.

However, the response of the caregiver needs to match the request. We don't all tolerate pain in the same way. If I don't want a painkiller – even though I say I'm in pain – that's my business.

O de G   The luck we have today is to have access to reliable sources of knowledge (books, networks, websites) that ensure everyone has access to information.

MW   Yes, there is no shortage of resources. And it's important to consult them, to understand what it means to be able to make informed choices when discussing something with a professional. To recognise 'bad practice' and not tolerate it. I often say that if you don't like what the doctor is suggesting, you can get up and leave – end of story. But in order to do that, you need to know what you need and what you don't need, to spend some time thinking about it.

SE   What would you recommend for reading around the subjects of bodies, sexualities and care?

MW   The first thing that springs to mind is *Our Bodies, Ourselves*, the book on female health that most influenced me when I was a student. The first American edition came out in 1970!

Witches, Midwives and Nurses, by Barbara Ehrenreich, and *Complaints and Disorders: The Sexual Politics of Sickness*, again by Barbara Ehrenreich and Deirdre English are two classics, both published in the 1970s. They describe in particular the discussions built up around women's bodies according to their social class, and how men took over the medical profession and marginalised them.

The Vagina Bible, by Jen Gunter, describes the physiology and ecology of the vagina with humour and anatomical precision. The work of a Canadian feminist woman doctor, at once scientific and full of common sense, this book sets straight all the myths and popular misconceptions about the vagina.

For a sociological description of the discrimination imposed by medicine on to women, there is a work by Caroline de Pauw, *La Santé des femmes* (Women's Health): it's very topical, well-researched and illuminating.

O de G   We would also like to recommend two of your works that convey your critical viewpoint of the behaviours of doctors and are essential reading: *C'est mon corps* (It's My Body), which explicitly responds in a practical way to the questions that women most frequently ask (themselves); and *Le Chœur des femmes* (The Women's Chorus), a novel you say was specifically written to bear witness to the abuse inflicted on women by doctors. It can be read as both a critical work and a self-defence or militant book in light of the brutality it details.

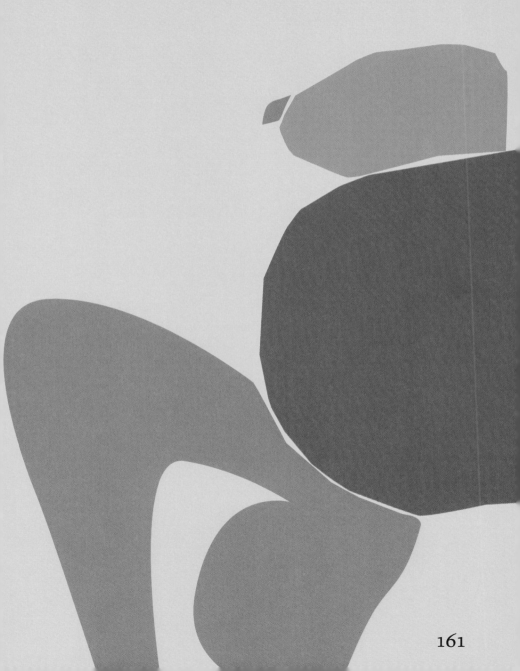

Chapter 9

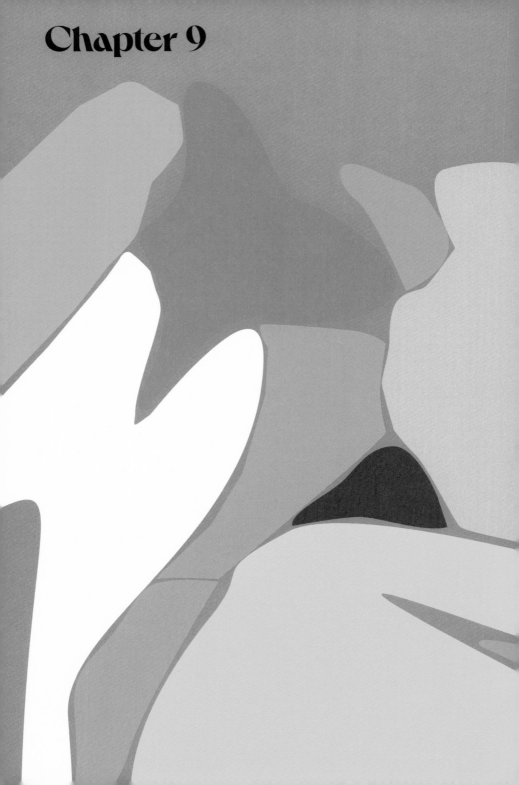

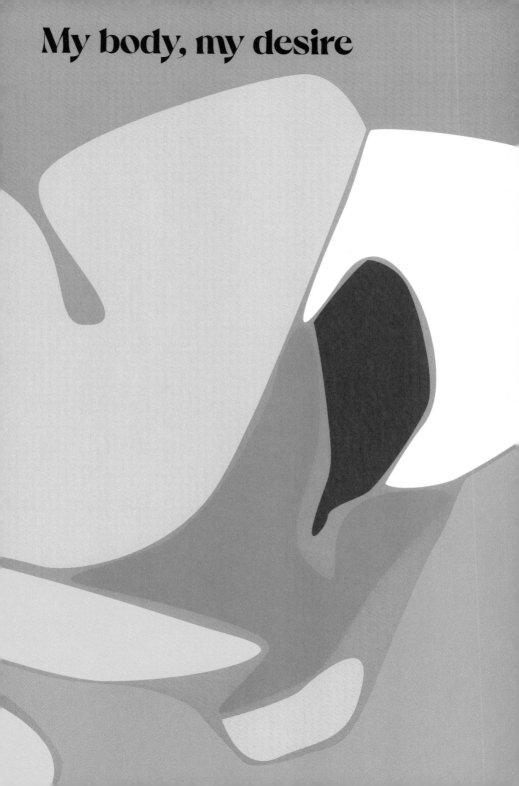

My body, my desire

And going forwards? How will I relate to my body, my desire?

When did it all tip over? When did I drop off the panel of women in whose company I'd have happily spent the whole evening? It's hard to say, exactly, but I get the impression my first pregnancy pushed me down the glamour list. I was thirty-five; my body very quickly filled out as an expectant mother, and I had to give up my combat trousers and tight T-shirts. And then, hallelujah, peace! No more comments from men in the street. Zilch. It was as though someone had cut off the torrent of garbage. It felt so good to be able to walk around freely, unhindered by having to anticipate a lewd comment, without fear of needing to respond: *No, not now, I don't want to, I can't, please FUCK OFF!*

'Drop-dead gorgeous', 'racy', 'shaggable'

However, along with the satisfaction of no longer being harassed, a new thought lodged itself in my brain: all this time, since I had first become aware of men's gazes on me (that is to say, from around the age of twelve!) until today, I had appeared in the public arena as a sexual object. I didn't live my life like that, of course, but it was part of what I was. Of what we were, us, young women. There is a sort of unspoken hierarchy: 'drop-dead gorgeous', 'racy', 'shaggable'. But even the latter attribution in this abject classification of the heteropatriarchy was imagined according to a status as a sexual object.

And since then? Since then, I've been invisible. Not least in the world of work. Once you're over forty-five or fifty, recognition comes to women only if they are already established, if they exist as a point of reference in some domain or another. If I were 'the architect who designed such-and-such a building', 'mayoress', 'editor-in-chief' or 'head of production', then I would have my place and the reassurance of recognition. For all those women – the majority – who are not top of these lists, it's a struggle to survive. Opportunities become ever scarcer; people don't immediately think of you when casting around, but of a man, or else a younger woman. This reality is well documented when you realise that in 2016, only 6 per cent of roles in French cinema went to female actors over fifty – whereas at the time, one adult woman in two was aged over fifty. Houdini couldn't have done it more skilfully: all you need to do is blow out that one extra candle on your birthday cake and – abracadabra! – you disappear.

Considering this, it's hardly surprising that so many women have a hell of a time looking to the future during their peri- and post-menopausal years. If we are invisible from the moment society no longer considers us as sexual objects, the margin for manoeuvre is incredibly narrow! Yet, you will say, cloaked in invisibility, we could do whatever we want: dye our hair blue or let it go silver, dance on tabletops until dawn, dress in low-cut clothes and wear monokinis on the beach with our sagging breasts, become a regular head-banger at heavy-metal concerts. And yes, of course, we could. But the looks, the comments, society as a whole, would condemn us, designate us as interlopers. Guilty of poor conduct. Our unfettered behaviour, removed from our roles validating us as women (sexual objects, fertile women, caregivers), renders us visible once more, for daring to exist outside our predestined path. We are openly defiant – we are witches. And by being so, we are exposing the dominant way of thinking.

All of which rather puts me in the groove to grow older...

More punk than elderly

If I'm honest, when I talk in this way – in lyrical-intellectual mode – it's generally when I've just had a fruitful discussion with my partner or with a girlfriend. Or read some pages from an uplifting and motivating book, such as the one by Mona Chollet. At the time of writing, I'm going through the stage of my life called the 'menopause'. An important turning point for which I was totally unprepared. My body is changing, but I'm not sure to what extent I want to welcome this new me. For the time being, I hardly have any white hairs, but what will I do in a while? Will I want to carry on being chestnut? Or, like my dear gynaecologist, will I dye my hair bright orange? Or will I leave my hair colour to take its natural course? And my body is thickening out: should I increase the amount of exercise I do, or just accept my more rounded figure?

Some mornings, when I catch my reflection in the bathroom mirror looking like an English bulldog, I'm scared I will no longer be able to seduce the man I love. That I'll be abandoned. Never be loved, ever again.

Some mornings, I rant and rave when confronted by the adverts framing my internet searches: 'How to firm up the skin on your neck if you're over fifty-five'; 'Stair lifts might be less of a luxury than you think'; 'You might be interested in these premium retirement apartments.'

Some mornings, I am irritated by reading the thoughts of well-meaning influencers who, by qualifying older women as 'grannies', relegate them to a perfectly idiotic role.

The documentary *Advanced Style* by Lina Plioplyte gives a voice to New York women over seventy who are super stylish in their physical approach to life, their choice of look – variously russet-haired with false eyelashes, gold-trimmed trousers, hats, bracelets, feathers, veils.

Once I'd got beyond the fascination of these elegant ladies and their joie de vivre, I realised that their prime message is badass before fashion. 'I do what I like.' That's what they are telling us. 'I know who I am and I look after myself, I'm the centre of attention wherever I go – and that's fine by me, thanks.'

So, some mornings, if I'm still raging inside about my ageing self, I remind myself of the magic formula: never let anything or anyone get between my desires and me; cultivate self-derision; rid myself once and for all of the standard exhortations (I don't give a toss about clothes sizes, I try on garments that might suit me); and leave space for what I like.

Today, I see the menopause as a sort of period of sloughing off, from which you can emerge with a new look, adorned for the next tranche of your life. That is to say: liking yourself. And even being attractive.

Industrial staircase and blow job

Olympe and I are due to meet in a town on the outskirts of Paris at the end of one of the Metro lines. It's dark. Two women are busy packing up a food truck on the square at the Metro station exit; further down the street, a bartender noisily pulls down the shutter. We follow the directions we received by email. We have to walk. The streets are empty. Not exactly the festive ambiance you'd choose when you're going out for the evening. On the opposite pavement, by way of reassurance, a group of people with coloured hair and carefully chosen clothes is heading in the same direction.

In the centre of an island of small brick houses – little courtyards and mini gardens and the usual clutter of children's toys, clothes lines, strings of material bunting, non-matching chairs and tables – it feels like we have, all of a sudden, been catapulted into a distant village.

> Perhaps we might be better off going back to the main road, suggests Olympe without taking her eyes off her GPS app.

But soon we're right behind the group with rainbow hair and some others, queuing in front of the small door in a huge entrance. A former factory. The doorkeeper who lets us in reminds us of the rules and regulations.

> It's not exactly Mitte, notes Olympe. But it's still fun to find ourselves in a sex- and body-positive environment.

Olympe is referring to the district in Berlin where the KitKatClub is located, a disco that opened in the 1990s and is famous for its sexual freedom and respect for all and sundry. Unlike the mythical club, access to this squat isn't purely reliant on looks, and there is a sense of freedom in seeing all these unclothed bodies, gyrating on the dance floor and round the bar.

Olympe gives me a signal and we go off to explore, each in our own direction. I climb an industrial staircase. The mezzanine is in partial darkness. It's warmer up here. Gradually, my vision adjusts to the low light. But I have difficulty believing my eyes. Olympe had warned me. Despite that,

I have to make an effort not to stare at the man kneeling in front of another man, giving him a blow job; or at these three women, dancing lasciviously while kissing and fondling each other. Other people are engaged in sexual activities, but not the majority. And most of all, those men and women who aren't thus occupied don't seem remotely bothered by those enjoying themselves. A bit like when the person you're sitting next to on the bus is watching a video of kittens on their phone; you straightaway know what it's about, and don't feel the need to keep staring at their screen.

Except, through habits of a lifetime, of course, I find it hard not to watch. So, rather than risk embarrassing anyone, I decide to go down to the landing below.

Fishnets, ponytails and wrinkles

The dance floor is packed. Arms waving in the air, bodies brushing past each other, people kissing, touching each other. There is a striking difference to other party venues I've been to in the past: here, there are all sorts of body types, bare-breasted, fishnet-stocking-hugged buttocks, long, hairy legs in high-heeled boots, a Goth-styled guy on walking sticks.

And then, quite quickly, I locate them: the older bodies I've secretly come to see. Olympe told me that this sort of event brings out all sorts of people, especially older ones. Not that there are crowds of them, but they are present, and that's what counts for me. In a chilled-out corner, half a dozen women, aged between sixty-five and seventy-five, in rock 'n' roll outfits – some of them in leather and jeans, one in full pin-up style, with a red gingham dress and her hair backcombed into a beehive – laugh, joke and kiss. A little way off the dance floor, a wiry man, bare-chested in knee-length cut-off jeans, dances despite evident weakness in his legs. And, sitting a couple of steps away from me on the staircase, a heterosexual couple hug each other. She has long grey hair tied up in a ponytail, her breasts erect under her vest; he has fuzzy white hair, a beard and a wizened face.

I went clubbing a couple of times during the 1990s. Bisexuals and homosexuals were able to find freedom on the club scene that was denied them elsewhere. Le Queen, Le Palace, El Hombre and Le Pulp... You could love there as you wished; you felt giddily light, giddily yourself. Although straight, I shared this sense of freedom with my mates, and felt cloaked in a gentle veil of foam, like when it's squirted on dance floors, and ready for some fast love.

Monogamy and the test of time

Full of enthusiasm, I tell Olympe about all the people with ageing bodies I've spotted. We smile.

> But if ageing bodily is one side of things, she picks up, there are also questions around sexual and loving relations. We become more and more demanding as we get older. And it can become hard to seduce. To be seduced. Sometimes I ask myself how I would cope if I found myself alone at seventy, but wanting some company.

When it comes to matters of seduction for those of advanced years, I always recall my elderly aunt, Simone. On the days she'd attend a dance, she would do her hair, slip into her most beautiful dress, and off she'd go. She must have been seventy when she came home with Léon, an adorable bear of a man with whom she set up home. They were 'good friends' as she called it.

> That's very sweet, says Olympe. For my part, I can't imagine being in a relationship where we are only 'good friends' like your aunt. Living with someone who doesn't desire me or, worse still, whom I don't fancy – that really doesn't appeal to me. Even if I imagine myself aged seventy-five.

> Hmmm... That opens up the question of monogamy and the test of time...

Sitting diagonally opposite me, and facing each other, the woman in red gingham and her female leather-clad friend, who a short while ago were crooning away, now appear deep in serious talk: hard-faced puppets with steely gazes whose body language screams mutual suspicion and even anger.

I like the idea of polyamory, Olympe continues. Reading *The Ethical Slut* made me want to try living in an open relationship. Building consensual, loving freedom with a partner. That's exactly the sort of life project I'd like to share: gradually forming, as time goes by, an open relationship between the two of us that suits both. That would allow us to avoid frustrations while still respecting the other person – other people.

I can't hide my grimace. At one point in time, I, too, considered polyamory. I felt a sort of pressure. All around me, everyone thinking about their lives seemed to be opting for polyamory. It appeared to be what you had to do in order for your couple to last: reflect, mature, remove any jealousy and prejudices; and accept sharing your lover(s).

I read the book by Dossie Easton and Catherine A. Liszt, along with blogs that touched on the same theme. To my great dismay, I had to accept that such a path was not for me. I found it hard to accept my inability to transform myself. I felt my own limits; I felt like a has-been. Idiotic.

But, with the passage of time, I have had the opportunity to re-think what I look for in love. I deconstructed this monogamy I had been indoctrinated with – and also the idea of heterosexuality. I questioned, once again, the ideas of polyamory, homosexuality, bisexuality, until I found myself facing a series of possible choices. It was no longer a question of doing what society expected of me, but rather what I wanted to do. What I really wanted was, 'simply', to be in a heterosexual, monogamous couple.

So, back to square one? Not exactly. Because I was making *my* choice from among a number of options. And I was doing so fully aware of the difficulties it entailed. Opting for monogamy means grasping *together* (which means being in agreement from the start) all those really annoying questions that you would rather brush under the carpet (not all at the same time, of course!): How do we ensure that daily life continues to be fun? How do we evolve sexually together? What ideas for the future do we have in common? How do we keep an open dialogue for the long term? How do we continue being curious about each other? How do we keep on renewing one another together – and not just on parallel tracks? How do I ensure that I remain aware of my desires, my needs? How do I share them with my partner? How do I make sure I'm available to listen to my partner's desires? How do we sustain them? How do we accept that there will be periods of isolation between us? And so on.

It's hard. But each milestone passed strengthens the link. Personally, I have enormous admiration for couples who, year after year, manage to put moments of crisis behind them, striking down the thousands of enemies that might have got the better of their determination.

When the summer draws to a close

On leaving the evening's festivities (my head still booming), I thank Olympe for this last exhilarating journey.

The body diversity, the joy, the sharing... All that is so good! We walk aimlessly, free as the wind.

We're at the end of our project, Olympe states. A year or so has passed and our investigation is drawing to an end.

I'm suddenly moved. We have dipped into vast numbers of books, discovered different points of view, confronted new perspectives, spoken with people who live these realities daily. Very different ourselves, we have always managed to exchange thoughts and understand each other. Perhaps because, as is the case for all women, the important thing is to identify what suits each of us individually, and to push away what oppresses us in our intimate sphere – whether we are twenty or sixty; whether lesbian, pansexual, asexual; whether militant feminist and ethical pornographer, or journalist-writer and mother.

There is one topic we haven't tackled, I say as we reach the food truck on the empty square.

If only there was just one ... Olympe says, with a smile.

The importance of education. The urgency with which we all watch children and adolescents growing up with their psychological and physical sensitivities. With their questioning about their bodies and their sexualities.

The taxi Olympe booked slows down beside us and parks up. She opens the door, I add:

We could even say that education and spreading information for each individual's enjoyment are the next huge tasks ahead...

I turn down Olympe's offer to drop me home. I feel like walking.

A dozen or so metres away, on the street leading back to the capital, I see two people, hand in hand. One in red gingham, the other in leather. They stop and kiss. They burst out laughing. A new day is about to dawn – for all of us. On the horizon, respectful and joyful love. Let us keep on moving forward.

Sources and Bibliography

Books, films, TV series... We are fortunate to live in an era in which questions of sexuality and our relationships with our bodies, while still being issues to defend, now occupy their own place in our daily lives. Each one of us can find areas for reflection according to our state of mind, our needs. Below, you will find the works mentioned in the book, as well as other titles we want to share because they have had an impact on our lives, our way of thinking – or simply because we were captivated by them.

Books (essays, cartoons, novels)

Atwood, M. 1985, *The Handmaid's Tale*, McClelland & Stewart, Toronto

Barker, M. J. & Scheele, J. 2016, *Queer: A Graphic History*, Icon, London

Beauvoir (de), S. 1949, *The Second Sex*, Gallimard, Paris

Bechdel, A. 2006, *Fun Home: A Family Tragicomic*, Houghton Mifflin Harcourt Publishing Company, Boston

Boston Women's Health Book Collective, The. 2011, *Our Bodies, Ourselves*, ninth edition, Simon & Schuster, New York

Brey, I. 2020, *The Female Gaze: A Revolution Onscreen*, L'Olivier, Paris

Černá, J. 1990, *Clarissa A Jiné Texty*, Concordia, Prague

Chollet, M. 2017, *Sorcières, la puissance invaincue des femmes* (Witches, the unvanquished power of women). Editions de la Découverte, Paris

Chollet, M. 2021, *Réinventer l'amour* (Reinventing Love), Editions La Découverte, Paris

Dennis, E. 2022, *Queer Body Power*, Jessica Kingsley Publishers, London

Despentes, V. 2010, *King Kong Theory*, Feminist Press, New York

Drouar, J. 2021, *Sortir de l'hétérosexualité* (Moving away from heterosexuality), Editions Binge, Paris

Easton, D. & Hardy, J. 2017, *The Ethical Slut: A Guide to Infinite Sexual Possibilities*, third edition, Ten Speed Press, Berkeley

Emmanuelle, C. 2016, *Sexpowerment, le sexe libère la femme (et l'homme)* (Sexpowerment, sex liberates women (and men)), Anne Carrière, Paris

Estournet, S. & de Gê, O. 2021, *Jouir est un sport de combat*, Larousse, Paris

Fazi, M. 2018, *Nous qui n'existons pas* (We don't exist), Dystopia Workshop, Paris

Feldman, D. 2012, *Unorthodox: The Scandalous Rejection of My Hasidic Roots*, Simon & Schuster, New York

Friedan, B. 1963, *The Feminine Mystique*, Norton & Co, New York

Fried-Filliozat, M. 2002, *L'Intelligence intime* (Intimate Intelligence), Robert Laffont, Paris

Froidevaux-Metterie, C. 2021, *Un corps à soi* (A body for itself), Seuil, Paris

Gallot, C. & Michel, C. 2020, *La charge sexuelle: désir, plaisir, contraception, IST... encore l'affaire des femmes* (Sexual Charge: desire, pleasure, contraception, STIs... still a woman's business), First Editions , Paris

Given, F. 2020, *Women Don't Owe You Pretty*, Cassell, London

Henning, A. M. & Bremer-Olszewski, T. 2012, *Make Love, Ein Aufklärungsbuch* (Make Love, An Education Book), Goldmann, Berlin

Hite, S. 1976, *The Hite Report*, MacMillan Publishing Co, New York

Illouz, E. 2018, *The End of Love: A Sociology of Negative Relations*, Suhrkamp Verlag, Berlin

Kirschen, M. 2021, *Herstory, Histoire(s) des féminismes*, Edition la Ville Brûle, Paris.

Maier, T. 2009, *Masters of Sex*, Basic Books, New York

Mermilliod, A. 2021, *Le chœur des femmes* (The Women's Chorus), Le Lombard, Brussels – a cartoon adaptation of Martin Winckler's eponymous novel

Moon, A. 2020, *Girl Sex 101, A Guide to Hot, Healthy Hook ups and Shame-free Sex*. Ten Speed Press, Berkeley

Nagoski, E. 2015, *Come as You Are*, Simon & Schuster, New York

Ngozi Adichie, C. 2018, *Dear Ijeawele, or a Feminist Manifesto in Fifteen Suggestions*, Harper Collins, New York

Page, M. 2020, *Au-delà de la pénétration* (Beyond Penetration), Le Nouvel Attila, Paris

Plã, J. 2020, Bliss Club, Hardie Grant Books, London

Preciado, P. 2010, *Pornotopía, Arquitectura y Sexalidad en Playboy durante la guerra fía,* (Pornotopia, Architecture and Sexuality in Playboy during the Cold War), Editorial Anagrama, Spain

Preciado, P. 2020, *An Apartment on Uranus: Chronicles of the Crossing*, MIT Press, London

Rubin, G. 2010, *Surveiller et Jouir, anthropologie politique du sexe* (Thinking Sex: Notes for a Radical Theory of the Politics of Sexuality), Epel, Paris

Shevchenko, I. and Hillier, P. 2017, *Anatomie de l'oppression* (Anatomy of Oppression), Seuil, Paris

Sontag, S. 1972, *Women and the Double Standard of Aging*, Women's Kit, Toronto

Sprinkles, A. 1998, *The Post Porn Modernist Manifesto*, Cleis Press, Minneapolis

Sprinkles, A, & Stephens, B. 2021, *Assuming the Ecosexual Position: The Earth as a Lover* (illustrations by Jennie Klein), University of Minnesota Press, Minneapolis

Strömquist, L. 2010, *Les Sentiments du prince Charles* (The Feelings of Prince Charles), Editions Rackham, Paris

Strömquist, L. 2016, *L'Origine de monde*, Rackham, Paris

Strömquist, L. 2018, *Fruit of Knowledge*, Virago, London

Taylor, S. R. 2018, *The Body is not an Apology*, Berrett-Koehler Publisher, Oakland

Tuaillon, V. 2021, *Le Cœur sur la table, pour une révolution romantique* (Your Heart on the Table, towards a Romantic Revolution), Editions Binge Audio, Paris

Valenti, J. 2008, *Yes Means Yes: Visions of Female Sexual Power and a World without Rape,* eds J. Friedman and J. Valenti, Seal Press, New York

Winckler, M. 2009, *Le chœur des femmes* (The Chorus of Women), P.O.L., Paris

Winckler, M. 2020, *C'est mon corps, toutes les questions que se posent les femmes sur leur santé* (It's My Body: All the Questions Women ask about their Health), Iconoclaste, Paris

Wittig, M. 1992, *The Straight Mind and Other Essays*, Beacon Press, Boston

Zeilinger, I. 2008, *Non, c'est non – Petit manuel d'autodéfense à l'usage de toutes les femmes qui en ont marre de se faire emmerder sans rien dire* (No Means No: A Pocket Self-Defence Manual for All Women Fed Up at Being Hassled But Not Responding), Éditions La Découverte, Paris

Films and TV Series

Ashford, M. 2013, *Masters of Sex*, Showtime

Blush, L. 2016, *Un beau dimanche*, Self-produced

Braeden Fox, S. 2017, *The 36-Year-Old Virgin*, A Beautiful Sunday

Cameron Mitchell, J. 2006, *Shortbus*, THINKFilm, Fortissimo Films, Q Television

Cohen, M. 2020, *I May Destroy You*, HBO

Dresen, A. 2008, *Septième Ciel* (Seventh Heaven), Rommel Film E.K

Dunham, L. 2012–2017, *Girls*, HBO

Gê (de), O. 2016, *The Bitchhiker*, Erika Lust Films

Gê (de), O. 2017, *Don't Call Me a Dick*, Erika Lust Films

Gê (de), O. 2017, *Take Me Through the Looking Glass*, Erika Lust Films

Gê (de), O. 2017, *We are the Fucking World*, Erika Lust Films

Gê (de), O. 2020, *Une dernière fois,* Canal Plus

Jouvet, E. & Delorme, W. 2010, *Too Much Pussy*, Womart Production

Kroll, N., Goldberg, A., Levin, M. & Flackett, J. *Big Mouth*, Netflix

Lee, S. 1986, *She's Gotta Have It*, 40 Acres & A Mule Filmworks, 1986.

Lee, S. 2017–2019, *She's Gotta Have It* (series), Netflix

Lust, E. 2017, *Architecture Porn*, Erika Lust Films

Manzoor, N. 2018–2022, *We Are Lady Parts*, NBCUniversal, Channel 4

Miller, B. 2017, *The Handmaid's Tale*, Hulu

Miller, B. 2018, *Female Pleasure*, Mons Veneris Films

Nolot, J. 2002, *La Chatte à deux têtes* (The Two-headed Pussy), Elia Films

Ovidie. 2017, *Pornocratie, les nouvelles multinationales du sexe* (Pornocracy, the new sex multinationals), Magnéto Press

Pelecanos, G. & Simon, D. 2017, *The Deuce*, HBO

Plioplyte, L. 2014, *Advanced Style*, Dogwoof

Saunders, J. & French, D. 1992–2012, *Absolutely Fabulous*, BBC2

Schrader, M. 2020, *Unorthodox*, Netflix

Soloway, J. 2014–2016, *Transparent*, Amazon Video

Soloway, J. 2016, *I Love Dick*, Amazon Video

Sprinkles, A. & Beatty, M. 1991, *How to Be a Goddess in 101 Easy Steps*, Self-produced

Waller-Bridge, P. 2016–2019, *Fleabag*, BBC Three

Online Resources

Advanced Style, www.advanced.style – women who age with elegance and tend to their looks, by photographer Ari Seth Cohen.

Cancer Rose, cancer-rose.fr – information on detecting breast cancer (in French).

ctrlX, ctrlx.fr – a platform offering audio creations developed from erotic and pornographic texts, co-created by Stéphanie Estournet (in French).

Les Fesses de la Crémière, *www.lesfessesdelacremiere. wordpress.com* – on open relationships and polyamory (in French).

Rupi Kaur, rupikaur.com – in 2015, the Canadian artist, Rupi Kaur, was censored by Instagram. The reason: her series *Period*, depicting menstrual blood.

Martin Winckler, www.martinwinckler.com – articles in French, English and Italian.

L'ecole des Soignant.e.s, ecoledessoignants.blogspot. com – a participatory and co-operative blog 'to put forward different teaching and care-giving models. To drill down into the ones that exist and deserve being reworked. To suggest and share other issues – whether ethical, practical, or sensitive – with today's and tomorrow's healthcare professionals' (in French).

Olympe de Gê, olympe-de-g.org/blog – Olympe de Gê's blog (in English and French).

OMGYes, www.omgyes.com: – 'The more you know, the better it is': this is the mantra of OMGYes. Aimed at everyone who is interested in female pleasure (in English and French; other languages available)

Shibari Study, www.shibaristudy.com – shibari tutorials carried out by experts (in English).

'Clitoris', *Thingiverse, www.thingiverse.com/thing:1876288* – the blueprint for a 3D clitoris designed by Odile Fillod (in English).

Voxxx, www.voxxx.org – audio-porn platform offering guided, immersive, inclusive and intimate masturbation sessions, co-created by Olympe de Gê (in English and French).

Platforms offering ethical, feminist and inclusive pornographic films

Bright Desire, brightdesire.com/tour
PinkLabelTV, pinklabel.tv

Make Love Not Porn, makelovenotporn.tv (amateur films)

TEDx Talks

Mintz, L. 2019, 'A New Sexual Revolution for Orgasm Equality', *TEDx*

Perel, E. 2013, 'The Secret of Desire in a Long-term Relationship', *TEDx*

Instagram accounts

@queen_esie – activist, artist and model, Esther Calixte-Bea celebrates the beauty of the body as it is.

@harnaamkaur – as someone with a hormonal imbalance, thirty-year-old activist, Harnaam Kaur, has decided to live with her beard (which she has nicknamed Sundry, meaning 'beauty' in Punjabi). She calls out harassment and encourages us to reflect on the image we have of ourselves and the models we are confronted with.

@meganjaynecrabbe – Megan Jayne Crabbe decided she'd had enough of all the nagging handed down to fat women to stay hidden or only show themselves if they were trying to lose weight. She wears bikinis, has pink hair and smiles at life.

Musical bonus

Bashung, A. 1991, 'Osez Joséphine'. Barclay/Universal, 1991
Hand Job Academy. 2014, 'Shark Week'. Independent

Pussy Riot. 2016, 'Straight Outta Vagina'. Big Deal / Nice Life / Federal Prism

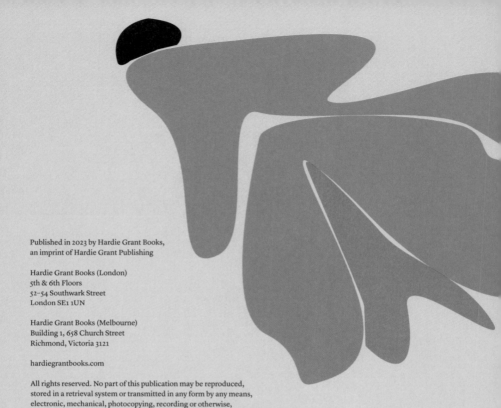

Published in 2023 by Hardie Grant Books,
an imprint of Hardie Grant Publishing

Hardie Grant Books (London)
5th & 6th Floors
52–54 Southwark Street
London SE1 1UN

Hardie Grant Books (Melbourne)
Building 1, 658 Church Street
Richmond, Victoria 3121

hardiegrantbooks.com

British Library Cataloguing-in-Publication Data.
A catalogue record for this book is available from the British Library.

Sex Talk
ISBN: 978-178488-442-0

10 9 8 7 6 5 4 3 2 1

Publishing Director: Kajal Mistry
Acting Publishing Director: Emma Hopkin
Commissioning Editor: Eve Marleau
Editor: Isabel Gonzalez-Prendergast
Copy Editor: Tara O'Sullivan
Proofread: Sophie Elletson
Art direction: Evi-O. Studio | Evi O.
Design & Illustrations: Evi O. Studio | Katherine Zhang
Production Controller: Gary Hayes

Colour reproduction by p2d
Printed and bound in China by Leo Paper Products Ltd.

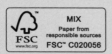